T0266995

Facial Reflexology
for Emotional Well-Being

"Having introduced a synthesis of Chinese and Ayurvedic medical approaches in my own work, I highly recommend Alex Scrimgeour's parallel integration of Vietnamese and Chinese medical approaches in *Facial Reflexology for Emotional Well-Being*. This outstanding book is a deeply thoughtful presentation of the history and practice of Vietnamese Dien Chan and its Chinese analogs that incorporate other styles of qigong. It is appropriate for both health care practitioners and the public at large."

PETER ECKMAN, M.D., PH.D., AUTHOR OF
THE COMPLEAT ACUPUNCTURIST

"Alex Scrimgeour beautifully weaves ancient wisdom with practical applications to help people connect with the cosmos and bring their spirit fully within. He eloquently describes the effective practice of Dien Chan that he studied with his master. This book makes a wonderful addition to the various self-care techniques that enhance the spirit and benefit the body's physiology."

CT HOLMAN, AUTHOR OF *TREATING EMOTIONAL*
TRAUMA WITH CHINESE MEDICINE

"This book is a treasure that not only shares the exquisite teachings of Dien Chan therapy but also takes us on a journey of holistic healing to our physical, emotional, and mental bodies."

JOVINNA CHAN, COFOUNDER OF THE
PRANOTTHAN SCHOOL OF YOGA

Facial
Reflexology
for Emotional
Well-Being

Healing and Sensory
Self-Care with Dien Chan

Alex Scrimgeour

Healing Arts Press
Rochester, Vermont

Healing Arts Press
One Park Street
Rochester, Vermont 05767
www.HealingArtsPress.com

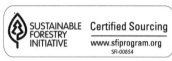

Text stock is SFI certified

Healing Arts Press is a division of Inner Traditions International

Copyright © 2023 by Alex Scrimgeour

All rights reserved. No part of this book may be reproduced or utilized in
any form or by any means, electronic or mechanical, including photocopying,
recording, or by any information storage and retrieval system, without permission
in writing from the publisher.

*Note to the reader: This book is intended as an informational guide. The remedies,
approaches, and techniques described herein are meant to supplement, and not to be a
substitute for, professional medical care or treatment. They should not be used to treat
a serious ailment without prior consultation with a qualified health care professional.*

Cataloging-in-Publication Data for this title is available from the Library of Congress

ISBN 978-1-64411-586-2 (print)
ISBN 978-1-64411-587-9 (ebook)

Printed and bound in the United States by Lake Book Manufacturing, LLC
The text stock is SFI certified. The Sustainable Forestry Initiative® program
promotes sustainable forest management.

10   9   8   7   6   5   4   3   2   1

Text design by Priscilla Harris Baker and layout by Virginia Scott Bowman
This book was typeset in Garamond Premier Pro and Futura with Palatino used as
the display typeface
Artwork by Kat Lowe

To send correspondence to the author of this book, mail a first-class letter to the
author c/o Inner Traditions • Bear & Company, One Park Street, Rochester, VT
05767, and we will forward the communication, or contact the author directly at
http:www.alexscrimgeour.com or **www.sensoryselfcare.com**.

Contents

List of Exercises

Healing Faces

Down a sleepy neighborhood alley in a busy part of Saigon, there lives an old man by the name of Dr. Tran Dung Thang. In all the street-side cafés and throughout the neighborhood he is well known and held in high esteem, for over the years he has brought relief and healing to many thousands of people. On a busy day he may treat up to one hundred people, despite the fact that he is well into his nineties. His wizened face, kind eyes, and long white beard lend him the air of an immortal sage straight out of a Taoist fairy tale. His bright mind, energy, and powerful voice all support this impression.

However, he is no mountain hermit and does not espouse any magical teaching. He is a man of the people and has lived in hectic Vietnamese cities all his life. He achieves his healing success with an unusual type of therapy—a unique system of Vietnamese facial reflexology called Dien Chan. From appearances, the way he works is by pressing and massaging different points and areas on the faces of his clients, using a variety of massage tools and a type of heat therapy called moxibustion.

On any given day, there is a queue of a dozen or so people waiting for treatment with him or one of his assistants. His studio is fully open to the street, which gives the whole atmosphere the feeling of welcome and friendliness. The people coming to see him are of all ages, from the very young to the elderly, and they suffer from every illness, pain, and disease you could imagine. The treatments are unique to each individual and last anywhere from five to ten minutes, at which point he playfully pretends to slap each patient, which without fail brings smiles and chuckles, and then sends them on their way. Treatment is based on donation, a gesture that reflects the ethos and compassion at the heart of both Dr. Tran and Dien Chan.

Having heard of his renown, I managed to track down the gentleman with the help of local friends, and when they discovered who he was they opted to receive treatment themselves. After three days of treatment my friend was greatly surprised to find that the nagging and painful tennis elbow he had been suffering from had completely disappeared! With some translation help, Dr. Tran welcomed me into his clinic to observe his treatments, where I passed many days absorbed in fascination and learning. This experience led me to enroll in one of his Dien Chan teaching courses. I was amazed by his boundless energy and deep compassion but equally puzzled by his treatments. This compelled me to search deeper into the nature and mechanics of Dien Chan, which in turn led me to delve into the holistic philosophy at the roots of traditional Asian medicine, the subtle dynamics between the face and body, between emotion and the nervous system, and eventually connected these to groundbreaking neuroscience that stands to shift our entire understanding of health and healing.

Through my journey I believe I have unveiled some of the hidden connections between the holistic healing traditions embodied in Dien Chan and the modern neuroscience and psychology of the face. This book is a way to share what I've learned and to help others benefit from both the treasure trove of traditional wisdom and the breakthroughs and innovations in contemporary health sciences.

◆ ◆ ◆

The human face is our most familiar image, it's the first thing we see when born, and in time, the faces we come to love are the deepest sources of joy and connection with the world. Unless we are a twin, the face we are born with is unique and tells a complex story of who we are, where we come from, and who we want to be. The face is a symbol of our humanity and reflects both who we are as a person and as a species. We have incredible nuance in our facial expression as a shape-shifting mask of communication and as a conduit for fully expressing and embodying our deepest delight.

The more you analyze the nature of the human face, the more layers are revealed. Our ancestry, upbringing, hardships, emotional trauma, temperament and character, kindness, hope, and wisdom—all of this can be revealed through the face, for one of our most innate evolutionary skills is to read one another's faces. To a greater or lesser degree, we are all experts at this, for our very survival depends on it.

This innate skill is part of what is called the social nervous system and operates largely below our conscious thinking mind. It is an instinct we are born with and gives us a split-second sense of who and what feels safe or dangerous. In turn, this cues our body to shift into a state of being at ease, which is essential for health and healing, or into a state of caution and alertness, which is essential for survival. Also known as the orientation mode of our nervous system, this distinctly human ability is so intrinsic that we are mostly unaware of it yet so patterned into our sense of self that it forms the bedrock of our worldview.

Our habitual facial expressions form the emotional template that governs whether we experience a healthy orientation response. The face carries an emotional weighting, which tilts our internal compass for navigating the dangers of life. Because of this it also plays a key role in health and well-being. What was once thought of as just a superficial aspect of the body, like an antenna to the world, is now known to be intimately connected to the deepest layers of both our physiology and psychology.

The face does not reflect just the mind, it is a physical parallel to our state of consciousness, so if our face is tense, our mind will be tense, too. This is a symbiotic relationship—when we relax our mind the face also relaxes, and when we release tension from the face, we also release the mind from tension and emotional stress.

Conversely, when we see people with a habitual flattening and hardening of the expression, particularly around the forehead and eyes, this often correlates with a history of suffering from trauma or depression. It's like a layer of emotional armoring has been created to buffer any future interactions that could be potentially painful. As the neurobiologist Stephen Porges says, "Faces become blank or flat when people become scared or challenged or are in pain."[1] This armoring also hampers our ability to mirror and empathize with other people and develop positive, nourishing relationships.

We all carry a degree of armoring; it's a natural human behavior to wear different masks to handle different situations, but unfortunately these masks sometimes become fixed, inhibiting our freedom and growth. If we physically wake up the face and reengage all the physiological structures and pathways, we can create a window of opportunity to break out of emotional patterns. This can be achieved from the outside in via Dien Chan self-massage or from the inside out by using the mind to internally engage with facial tension and our sense organs.

We now know that there is a strong link between emotional and physical pain, as they appear to light up the same pathways in the brain.[2] The scientific study of pain, like emotion, is currently experiencing a paradigm shift, which is slowly filtering into mainstream medicine and therapy. Some researchers even describe pain as an emotion. Although I don't believe the phenomena of emotional or physical pain can be entirely reduced to brain physiology, Dien Chan seems to be tapping in to these pathways where physical and emotional healing are intertwined. Whether we suffer physically or emotionally, the expression on our face is of the same dynamic, and this illustrates the deep entanglement between our physicality and our consciousness.

Of course, it is not just the face that is entangled in this dynamic, the whole body is, too. Our emotions can be felt just as strongly in our chest, belly, or face. It just so happens that the face is uniquely positioned to change our sensorial experience as well as our perception of the world around us. It is for this reason, that if we can change the relationship we have with our face, we can in turn change the relationship we have with the world.

Dien Chan therapists like to describe the face as a master control panel for all the physiological and mental-emotional processes of the body. I would take it further and suggest that the face contains a profound ability to reconfigure our entire relationship with the world around us.

By increasing our moment-to-moment awareness of our face we can begin to map out the layered connections that cascade through our nervous system, breathing and heartbeat, emotions and feelings, right down to the piezoelectric charge in our bones. This process begins with igniting a curiosity toward the nature of our sense organs and a willingness to question our senses. We form a question not with our words or even our thoughts but at the most bare-naked level—at the level of feeling. When we feel into the body, rather than searching for an answer, we are simply open to feeling what is there, a neutral listening under the skin. In meditation this is sometimes called inner hearing or inner vision; in neuroscience this is called interoception and refers to a very real sense we have that is distinct from the typical five senses.

By developing this felt sense of the body we are also developing our capacity to change our relationship with the body. If we remain in a state of calmness and safety as we explore the interoceptive space of our body, this will soothe and re-pattern our nervous system, which can heal both chronic pain and emotional trauma. We can't change what we can't feel, or as James Baldwin said, "Not everything that is faced can be changed; but nothing can be changed until it is faced."[3]

If we can feel how the tension around our eyes or in our throat connects to the more subtle internal sensations of our emotions, mood, and temperament, we can start to grasp how much our biology drives us. We can start to see how our habitual reactivity and biological stance twists our perception of the world. If our social nervous system is orientated toward being on the defensive, for instance, then this will change how we see and hear other people and what we notice in the world around us.

However, if we can retain a curiosity and openness in our orientation, then we can initiate a type of inquisitive alchemy, wherein the very act of paying attention to our perception transmutes it. Henry Corbin famously stated that "alchemy is the sister of prophecy."[4] The prophetic referred to here does not mean to speak of what will become but rather is pointing toward our awakening and more awakened ways of perception. So, by re-patterning our senses we engage in a type of alchemy, one that transforms old patterns of self-deception, rewires our physiology, and forges new ways of being in the world. The metaphorical gold we produce is the experience of perpetually awakening to a more vivid and truthful beholding of the world.

This is where the practice of Dien Chan connects with the meditative and contemplative arts. Not only does Dien Chan offer a system of wellness, radical self-care, and healing, but it also offers itself as a kind of psychotechnology that can keep our senses lucid and clear. Dien Chan directly engages our sense perception and the structures of our social orientation system, therefore offering us a tool for guarding ourselves from self-deception as well as a way of learning to make sense of the world with more clarity and discernment. In the era of post-truth and the attention economy, our senses are hyperstimulated and overstrained. I believe the methods and techniques of Dien Chan can greatly support us in navigating our way forward.

However, rather than frame it as some kind of magic bullet that will solve all our woes, it is better seen as a single thread in a woven ecology of practices. Breathwork, exercise, diet, sleep hygiene, meditation, contemplation, and the social nourishment of friendship, music, and ritual are just as important in an ecology of practice. The beauty of Dien Chan is that it's like a keystone in this ecology—it can interface between our internal and external worlds, enriching all these life habits and bridging the embodied self with the external world. It can help us feel embedded and in kinship within our community and within nature as a whole. In other words, it works on both the personal, communal, and ecological levels.

My personal story of how I came to discover this practice is one of curiosity, luck, and good fortune. When we are young our minds are wide open and naïveté is our great strength, for it multiplies all the possibilities of the world. When I was on the cusp of growing out of childhood, as my opinions and worldview were beginning to take shape, I discovered a great love—books. As chance would have it, one particular book landed on my lap that would set off a chain of events that led me to my path. It was a book of fiction, written by an anthropologist, about the initiation of a boy into the arts of the shaman and set in premedieval England, the country of my birth. It gave me a glimpse of a different way of seeing the world, one that is collaborative in nature rather than one of control and domination.

This book sparked a curiosity that drew me into avidly reading all I could about what we call shamanism, the prereligious mode of spirituality that guided our ancestors for the majority of human history. I read all of Carlos Castaneda's books with gleeful naïveté before I was sixteen. I became privately obsessed with all that pushes the limits of the imagination, esoteric systems and heretic beliefs, and all that the modern West tends to sneer at and rejects as reeking of magic.

I became fascinated with indigenous cultures precisely because they offered something that was abysmally lacking in modern culture. It wasn't just the sense of intimate human community that you see in village life, or the feeling of belonging to the natural world and not vice versa. It was a lost mode of being—an entirely different way of standing in the world that is mostly seen in the stance and speech of the shaman. It is also present in one form or another throughout the great spiritual traditions of the world. I have explored many of these wisdom traditions and still find it incredible that we have access to such a treasure trove of old teachings, from Buddhism, Daoism, Vedanta, Sufism, African, and Mesoamerican cultures, and even indigenous European folk traditions.

It's a curious thing how so many of these lineages have remained secret for generations, and only in the past fifty years or so there's been this grand disclosure. I suspect there is a deeper significance to this beyond simply the rise of the internet and the homogenization of culture. When these old lineages are exposed to one another there is an interesting cross-pollination that takes place, and great potential arises.

In any case, I had the good fortune to learn with many skilled teachers, healers, shamans, and mystics. Some of the most profound teachings I was exposed to did not originate from the teacher or tradition themselves but rather through the shift in attention encouraged by the teacher to learn directly from both my intrinsic nature and from the natural world itself. As such, the teaching is often not a specific knowledge but points to a way of listening, a way of being acutely receptive to the world. This is an entirely different approach from what is taught at most schools or universities; it is a different type of knowledge, a way of knowing that participates with the world in real time. It is what the Greeks called *anagoge,* a way of knowing that creates a transparency between the mundane and the sacred—that keeps one ear alert to what is and one ear alert to what might be. This is particularly apparent in the witnessing of nature's splendor and beauty. Partly because of my love of nature, I found myself fascinated by and resonanating with Daoism, the indigenous philosophy of China and perhaps the longest standing of the great traditions.

The roots of Daoism lie in a shamanic culture that predates the second millennium BCE, evolving gradually into both a religious practice and a system of thought that underpins Chinese civilization. It offers a comprehensive philosophy of nature and our place within it.

The wonderful thing about Daoism is that it breaks out of the books and can be experienced vividly through a culture of embodiment practices. It offers a great deal to the intellect, but subversively, it also offers a way to engage the body, shifting our intellect in unexpected directions. These mind-body practices have in modern times come to be called qigong. It was these practices that most tangibly brought my exploration of the written word into the real world. After many years of practice, qigong and meditation became a greater and greater part of my life, so I naturally sought to find a way to make them a part of my livelihood. I wanted to spend all my time immersed in this way of life. This led me to studying acupuncture and Chinese medicine* as a full-time degree, which initiated me into an entirely different way of understanding health and seeing our place in the world.

I was also lucky enough to have a mentor through this degree,

---

*Throughout this book you will see the terms *Chinese medicine, Traditional Chinese Medicine,* and *Classical Chinese Medicine.* Traditional Chinese Medicine and Classical Chinese Medicine have notable differences, particularly in their use in this book, as does the more general Chinese medicine. Traditional Chinese Medicine refers to specific forms of Chinese medicine that were systematized by the communist restructuring of China in the 1950s, whereas Classical Chinese Medicine describes a style that is not as modernized and adheres more closely to the classical texts of Chinese medicine. The term *Chinese medicine* in this book is being used as a general term for medicine in China versus a specific system.

whom I shadowed for a number of years in his clinical practice. It was he who sent me out to Vietnam to gain clinical experience in the main acupuncture hospital of Ho Chi Minh City. Often people question why I didn't go to China to learn, and the answer is complex. Vietnam has a long and turbulent history with China, having even been conquered at one point and consequently ruled by China. There is a big Chinese cultural influence in Vietnam, particularly in Buddhism, Daoism, and Confucianism, but there is also very distinct indigenous Vietnamese culture and medicine. There is a shared source in the ancient classical texts of Chinese medicine, but there are also styles of healing that are uniquely Vietnamese.

Historically the Chinese emperor and ruling class sought to create a uniformity in belief and custom, with gradual stages of standardization in medicine. People who went against the grain were often banished from the kingdom and sent south, away from the capital, often ending up in Vietnam. For this reason, Vietnam absorbed a lot of the outlier and unusual medical practices. Combine this with the strong local animist traditions and the result is a melting pot of innovation and generally a more open-minded approach to healing.

So, studying in Vietnam can be a more interesting experience, as the tendency in China since the Communist revolution has shifted toward a more generic, less nuanced style of practice.

It was during my time spent in Vietnam that I heard about this unusual form of therapy in which practioners were treating only the face achieving remarkable results. I experienced a treatment myself and realized this was very different from any type of reflexology or massage I'd ever had. The fact that it was so popular in Vietnam but quite unknown outside of the country also intrigued me. I began a personal study of this system, which brought me back to Saigon every year to learn, exploring the different styles and approaches of various Dien Chan specialists.

Because of my background in acupuncture and Chinese medicine,

I was able to cross-reference the Dien Chan approach and place it within the greater context of Classical Chinese Medicine. During this same period, I was also moving toward specializing in stress and trauma, a field that is experiencing a renaissance that I believe will have serious implications for healthcare in general. I spent several years teaching qigong and serving tea ceremony in a residential clinic specializing in trauma recovery. As these different strands of knowledge came together, I began to see some fascinating connections between the Dien Chan treatments I was giving and their context within the fields of trauma and Classical Chinese Medicine. This new way of understanding the nervous system and its primary importance in the dynamics of stress and trauma ties right into facial reflexology and its development in Vietnam in the wake of the Vietnam War. The vast majority of patients who were initially being treated were undoubtedly suffering from the trauma of the war to one degree or another, particularly as one of the first places it was trialed in was an addiction clinic.

There is an even greater parallel if we consider the history of qigong and its roots in Classical Chinese Medicine, philosophy, and shamanism. A major factor in PTSD (post-traumatic stress disorder) and stress is that our senses begin to deceive us—we see and hear danger where there is none. By directly working with the senses, we can begin to reset our perception back to a clearer picture of reality. Both Dien Chan and qigong have a strong ability to affect the senses in this way, as both engage our sense organs in novel ways.

The body expresses the effects of trauma in unusual ways. It can create a masking effect over the face, but more systemically it can give a sense of entrapment in the body, a feeling of both being trapped in the body and of having something pernicious trapped in one's body. It can also feel as if one is trapped out of the body and cannot fully inhabit it. The natural way that the body expresses and releases these feelings often results in the phenomenon of physical trembling and shaking, which occurs in the immediate wake of trauma and also in the therapeutic regulation of the nervous system. Although when the body spontaneously begins trembling this might seem unusual or even scary, it is now known that this can be a natural and healthy response, particularly when there is a preestablished sense of safety. It is a way for the nervous system to discharge the extreme tension and stress that the body is put under during traumatic or overwhelming events.

This spontaneous trembling can be facilitated by certain qigong techniques, and curiously I also began noticing my clients release tension in this way during Dien Chan treatments. There is always the same effect after this happens—a sense of deep relaxation and increased contentment in the body.

One of the beautiful things about Dien Chan and qigong is that they are relatively easy to learn and apply on oneself. They awaken your own healing power and put it in your own hands. However, the more we understand the context of where they come from and the principles that are at play, the more we will empower ourselves and realize the potential for transformation. It is one thing simply to know a certain technique, but if we have a clearer understanding of why we are doing it then this brings with it a richer experience, with a greater clarity of intent, that will affect a deeper change.

For this reason, we will explore the background of Classical Chinese Medicine, qigong, shamanism, and Daoist philosophy. For the same reason, we will look at innovations in neurobiology and the implications these have for understanding stress, trauma, the nature of consciousness, and our general health and well-being. Along the way I will introduce various techniques that you can learn, which will give you a tangible feel and appreciation for both the philosophical principles and psychoneurological dynamics at play. These exercises and techniques stem from Dien Chan and my training in qigong, meditation, and Chinese medicine. I encourage you to remain open-minded and to seek the natural enjoyment that arises as you get a feel for these practices.

USING THIS BOOK

I've written this book primarily to share the Dien Chan and qigong self-care practices that are so helpful for mental, emotional, and physical health. These techniques can be learned, practiced and taught by just about any person. They are relatively simple, and it would be difficult to do anything wrong. At the worst, inattentiveness might lead to scratching yourself or poking yourself in the eye! This is quite unlikely, though it should be emphasized that mindfulness and attentiveness are the best guides to finding the correct pressure. Mindfulness of the body as we practice self-massage is a vital part of the therapeutic effect.

Generally speaking, the contraindications for self-treatment pertain more to the use of massage tools and the more applied pressure they create. I recommend that anyone who is pregnant should avoid the space between the nose and upper lip, which when pressed with force can risk stimulating contractions.

For all these exercises we simply use our hands and nothing else. If you have dry skin, feel free to use a little skin oil or cream, but not too much as we need a certain amount of traction for many of these techniques to work well. For those who are interested in going further into tools and point protocols look to appendix A, which introduces tools for going deeper into this practice.

There are a couple of comprehensive textbooks and some well-produced mobile apps that list the main point protocols, and I would recommend exploring these if, say, you're looking for a specific protocol for a health ailment. As a starting point I would go to the Dien Chan FACEASiT app or Marie-France Muller's classic book, *Facial Reflexology: A Self-Care Manual.* My intention for this book is to focus on learning how to switch our body more broadly into the healing mode. The real power of Dien Chan as a therapy lies not in finding the precisely located point but in finding what is called the living point. This means finding the areas and points on the face that have a particular sensitivity to them. And this can only be done by feeling, listening inside, and becoming familiar with the overarching principles.

Therefore, this book both sets the stage for further explorations and for understanding the deeper layers and dimensions of the face. It is specifically geared toward emotional well-being and working with stress and trauma. However, the great majority of all health and emotional problems are deeply connected to stress and trauma, and so this book is intended to help as broad an audience as possible. With greater insight into the dynamics of the face, this practice can also be used for self-inquiry, meditation, and for exploring the deeper mechanisms of perception and aesthetics. Hopefully by the end you will feel confident that you can use these principles and techniques to tailor your own self-care treatments and be rewarded with the benefits.

The framework I use is not strictly how Dien Chan is taught in Vietnam or how acupuncture or qigong are taught in China or the West. I take a very wide-angle approach to these practices, which draws from both the long and diverse histories of Dien Chan, qigong, and trauma as well as my personal experience and understanding of traditional medicine, meditation, and the modern scientific insights into trauma therapy, stress, and consciousness.

Traditionally, Chinese and East Asian medicine have been pluralistic, meaning that there is not one standardized approach but rather a multitude of approaches that correspond to the specific environment and climate of the doctor, the doctor's philosophical and technical disposition, and the field of expertise in which they find themselves. I carry on this approach by respectfully adapting and innovating to best match what I see as most pressing in our modern times.

Because of this wide-angle approach, we explore the history of these practices in chapters 1 through 3 to give a fuller context for how these traditions have developed. In chapters 4 through 13 we gradually uncover the different aspects of our face and the various principles and techniques that can catalyze positive change and healing.

The core practical exercises, which are contained in chapters 7, 9, 11, and 14, are designed specifically toward changing our relationship with stress and creating a feeling of being balanced and calm in mind and body. The final two chapters turn toward using Dien Chan in combination with meditative practices. These chapters are intended to be approached after establishing the core practices, for they work in a more subtle way with our sense perception.

Feel free to skip straight to the practical chapters if you want to dive straight in. However, the structure of the book is designed to slowly introduce you to why and how these practices work, and this can both heighten our appreciation for what we are doing and focus our intention on it. As we move into the later chapters, we will see that our mental state and intention play an important role in Dien Chan.

Although these practices hold great potential for our physical, mental, and emotional health, I recommend that you frame them within an ecology of practice. This means they are best used alongside a healthy lifestyle, and as a supportive adjunct to personal routines, whether it be exercise, meditation, yoga, cooking, self-inquiry, or within our social rituals. If you are in the midst of trauma or coping with integrating PTSD symptoms, I recommend you seek support from your social circles and from appropriate health workers. The techniques in this book can be a powerful support for those with trauma but, as mentioned earlier, shouldn't be taken as a magic bullet. Rather, they offer us a helping hand toward the first step in recovering from trauma or dealing with stress, both of which depend on establishing a sense of safety. Through Dien Chan we can also develop a more tangible understanding of our nervous system and our mind and move toward what I call an orientation toward beauty.

Finally, I have created an online companion video course that gives you live demonstrations of the practices and techniques in this book. It can be found at www.sensoryselfcare.com. Depending on your style of learning, you may find it easier to practice alongside these videos, as they offer more detail for the specifics of each massage. However, hopefully you will find the outlined descriptions in this book sufficient, because I have endeavored to make them as simple, clear, and accessible as possible.

. . . .

ONE

The Roots of Dien Chan Facial Reflexology & Qigong

DIEN CHAN IN HISTORY AND CONTEXT

Dien Chan was first developed in the late 1970s by Professor Bui Quoc Chau, a distinguished Vietnamese doctor who was working at that time in an addiction clinic in Ho Chi Minh City.

Vietnam was still reeling from a devastating war and many decades of repression under colonial France. On top of this, a communist revolution was upending the traditional culture and way of life. In short, it was a hard time and place to be alive.

No doubt the reason most people found themselves suffering from addiction was not due to any moral failing but rather a dire need for some kind of coping mechanism for dealing with the trauma of these times. As is the case with the majority of addictions, the root cause lies in one's response to trauma and/or childhood adversity. But at this time, PTSD wasn't yet recognized, and the means of treating addiction and trauma were undeveloped. For this reason, Bui Quoc Chau found himself innovating to try to find new ways to help his patients.

He was trained in acupuncture and discovered that using needles on specific points on the face would unexpectedly create positive results, and not just with addiction but also with different types of pain and illness. From his knowledge of traditional medicine, ancient philosophy, and modern physiology, he developed a new therapeutic model, one that could address all manner of health problems without the need for drugs or surgical intervention but instead by simply using the medium of the face.

One of his key innovations was the realization that he didn't need acupuncture needles to achieve good results—the sensitivity of the face was such that using a small massage tool would suffice. This made the treatment much more accessible, as using many needles on the face can be intense and overwhelming. It also led to the creation of many specially designed massage tools that could stimulate and affect the face in different ways.

If we consider the traditional functions of the acupuncture points that cover the face, you will find they are typically used to treat the senses and sense organs, to treat headaches, or to affect the mind. There are many acupuncture points on the body that also affect the head and senses. For example, there are points on the hands that relieve headaches and on the feet that treat tinnitus. What Bui Quoc Chau discovered was that the opposite is also true, that there are points on the face that can heal things such as wrist pain, breathing issues, and even edema in the legs.

Over a long period of experimentation, he mapped out more than three hundred specific points on the face, each with unique functions and healing potentials. Although he took into consideration the network of acupuncture channels and secondary branches that cover the face, his main reference for discovering the nature of these points was in superimposing different images of the body onto the face. This is the same method you see in foot reflexology, wherein the organs and anatomy of the body are overlaid onto the sole of the foot, and by treating the associated area on the foot, the body can be prompted toward healing. This is why Dien Chan is translated as "facial reflexology."

However, in Dien Chan there isn't just one image but more than twenty different images that are overlaid onto the face. For this reason, it is sometimes called multireflexology, as this is a feature unique to Dien Chan and hints at the dynamic principle that it's guided by. This principle stems from an older source in ancient Chinese philosophy— the concept of *ganying*. This term is often translated as "resonance" or "corresponding resonance," as it refers to the way in which things of similar form naturally vibrate, syncopate, and harmonize with one another. It can be observed not only through human life but throughout the natural world as well. It is a universal principle that both predates and informs the foundational pillars of Classical Chinese Medicine, yin-yang theory, and five element theory. These theories give structure to and systematize this principle of ganying.

For example, in the old medical texts it is said that the ears and sense of hearing correspond with the kidneys. At first blush this might seem bizarre, as these two parts of the body are so different. However, if we look at embryological development, we will see that both the kidneys and ears uniquely develop from the same tissue source in utero.[1] This tells us that they do indeed have a shared origin and connection. In five element theory, the water element brings together many disparate aspects of the body and the world, including the kidneys, ears, sense of hearing, bones, bladder, the emotion fear, the season winter, the color blue, and the taste of salt. All these things are thought to share a connection through ganying and therefore have an ability to resonate and influence each other. For this reason, acupuncture points relating to the kidney meridian are often used for problems relating to the ears and hearing, as they share a corresponding resonance and can affect one another.

Dien Chan has flipped this corresponding relationship and, for example, uses points around the ears to affect the health of the kidneys and adrenals. At some level, the mechanism behind this could be thought of as stemming from the embryological development of the nervous system and a phenomenon of anatomical mirroring that occurs in the brain. However, the concept of ganying suggests a much broader perspective, one that says that at the most fundamental level of our bodies and of all reality, there is a holographic and interdependent nature. This means every single part of our body contains a reflection of the whole. It also means that each reflection of the whole contains an image not just of our physicality but also of our consciousness, for the mind and body are united in our sense of wholeness.

Dien Chan has discovered that within the human face there are many, many reflections of the whole. By using the resonant properties of the body, Dien Chan can harmonize many aspects of our health and, more significantly, can shift us toward a state of wholeness. Professor Bui explored the vast amount of facial interconnections and created new maps that detailed how specific points and areas on the face affect all aspects of our physiology. There are more than three hundred points mapped on the face alone. He helped countless people not only as a healer but also as a teacher, for Dien Chan can be learned by any person who wishes to harness their own intrinsic power for self-healing.

Over the years Dien Chan grew to become an incredibly popular therapy and spread throughout Vietnam. The main reasons for this are because it is effective, relatively easy to use, and inexpensive. Although there are now many teachers and clinicians, the therapy is still relatively unknown outside of Vietnam. This is similar to much of Vietnamese traditional medicine and to Vietnamese culture in general, which is usually eclipsed by pop culture references to the Vietnam War.[2]

Although intellectually it might be fairly easy to grasp the idea that everything is interconnected and in resonance, at its inception thousands of years ago, ganying emerged from a culture and worldview that was drastically different from and in contrast with our present times.

Therefore, to really grasp this idea we have to extend our imaginative reach, we have to envision what the world might have seemed like for someone living five thousand years ago.

QIGONG IN HISTORY AND CONTEXT

Qigong has a much older history than Dien Chan and lies at the core of Classical Chinese Medicine—it literally embodies the cosmology that underpins Chinese culture.

The word *qigong* is actually an umbrella term used for a wide array of traditional Chinese and East Asian mind-body practices. For the past three thousand years these practices have been developing and evolving in response to the cultural changes of China, particularly in relation to health and medicine, religion, and martial arts. Combining aspects of meditation with exercise and self-massage, qigong has spread to the West over the past forty years, and now new forms of qigong have even emerged from Western masters. Qigong does not refer to a single agreed upon practice but instead is inclusive of many contrasting therapeutic, martial, gymnastic, mythotheatric, and spiritual arts. There are literally thousands of styles and forms, all with slightly different objectives and methodologies. For this reason, it is often misunderstood, misinterpreted, and underestimated when considered without its full historical context.

There is both a modern context, which has had a fascinating and turbulent history in the past few hundred years, and an ancient context, which relates more broadly to the development of Daoism and the birth of Chinese civilization. Although we have good documentation of the more recent changes in the qigong field, the further we go back in time the less clear things become. Much has been lost and can only be speculated upon. One reason is that some lineages are only passed down orally. Another reason is that the old writings and books have perished, most noticeably in the book burnings that occurred in the first century BCE. And yet another reason is that the roots of qigong lie so far back that they parallel the roots of writing itself. At its inception, Chinese writing was originally a form of mediumship between the spiritual planes—only later did it grow beyond the bounds of oracles and become a tool for human communication.

However, some things we can be more sure of. Qigong developed out of shamanic practices that sought kinship with all the natural world. Some of these practices included shape-shifting and mimicked the movement and gestures of animals. Some sought to enter learning partnerships with plants, herbs, and trees and formed the phenomenological basis of herbal medicine. Some sought to enter into deeper relationships with the greater spheres of the natural world, with the sun and moon, with stars, with mountains and rivers, and with the elemental natures of fire and water.

The people who were most astute at these practices were those who could walk easily between the human and nonhuman worlds. This is outside the realm of logic and reason; it is a rare transcendent apprehension of our being and the world around us—a heightened sensitivity to the processes we are embedded in and also the processes that are embedded in us. To transcend and see through our own humanity is actually quite a terrifying thing, and so shamans of all ilk have a tendency to be on the outskirts of society, at the edges of the village, or in many cases, living solitarily in the great mountains. This is where qigong has its historical birthplace—not in the valleys and planes, but closer to heaven, in the mountains.

As these practices became more established and interfaced with the wider society, they began to align with the philosophy and culture that developed in the golden age of Chinese antiquity, the Zhou Dynasty period, during which time it is said that one hundred schools of thought blossomed. We can trace the earliest copies the Dao De Jing and the Yi Jing, the classic books that seeded the formation of Daoist philosophy and Confucian culture to this period. Both of these books looked to nature and its cycles and patterns as sources of wisdom and intelligence. Rather than separating and elevating human intelligence as supreme, these texts described human intelligence and human virtue as being embedded in and arising from a greater field of intelligence and virtue inherent in the natural world.

At the core of this belief lies not an intellectual certainty but a knowing of the heart and the gut, an experiential connection that supersedes linear, objective understanding. This way of connecting to the world through the totality of our felt experience was a guiding light for the emergence of Daoism and Classical Chinese Medicine. And this way of connection has in modern times come to be known as qigong.

Qigong is most closely associated with the philosophy and religious practices of Daoism but over the centuries has blended with Confucian principles, Buddhist thought, and even Christianity and Islam. It is as much a spiritual psychotechnology as it is a physical exercise. It forms the bedrock of many medical practices and is the secret power to many systems of martial arts. It has evolved and changed over the centuries and more recently has undergone some extraordinary developments.

Qigong, in parallel with the recent history of Daoism and Traditional Chinese Medicine, has seen great upheaval and disaster in the past hundred years. It's very lucky that these ancient practices have survived at all. The first wave of adversity was brought by Western influence, in the forms of a new paradigm-shaking ideology and science, and then by colonial forces that crippled the country and helped bring the downfall of the last emperor.[3] The second wave came after World War II and the Chinese Civil War, as the communist revolution purged the country of anything that was connected to the old culture. Chinese medicine itself was unsuccessfully banned for a few years earlier in the century and was nearly outlawed by the communists. However, they saw a great opportunity in traditional medicine due to both its efficacy and low cost. The only downside was its connection to Daoism and traditional culture. So, in the 1950s the Communist Party completely revised how Chinese medicine was practiced so that it could be integrated with Western medicine, administered effectively in hospitals, and taught en masse in universities.[4] Prior to this it was only practiced in family-run clinics and passed down in family lineages through strict apprenticeships which meant the whole field had thousands of different contrasting approaches and theories, and by its nature was pluralistic.[5] Chinese medicine readily accepted that two contrasting theories could be equally valid and effective, that there are different orders of truth that can encapsulate the workings of human health.[6] But in the 1950s it was standardized and regulated in a way that simplified complex skills and stripped away anything connected to Daoism and spirituality, including the emotional and spiritual components of the medicine, which are actually at its core.

At this same time, medical qigong was formalized and the first qigong hospitals were created in which qigong healing was given alongside many hours of daily qigong practice. This was a very interesting period that was unfortunately halted in the late 1960s with the humanitarian disaster known as the Cultural Revolution, an incredibly traumatic time during which it is estimated that millions of people died due to a combination of famine, violence and murder, and a complete breakdown of bureaucratic, social, and health care services. In the aftermath, Chinese society was tyrannized and oppressed, with very limited individual freedom. But a strange twist of fate led to a resurgence of qigong during this time.

It was said that a high-ranking Chinese Communist Party member was cured of a life-threatening illness by a certain qigong master, and for this reason the practice of qigong had official sanction. And so, qigong became the only public activity where people could come together in groups, socialize outside of their government units, and learn this healing art.[7] Not only did it represent an exception to extreme social oppression, but it also offered a form of catharsis and healing from the horrors of the previous decade.

This strange situation led to what is known as qigong fever, where millions of people suddenly became obsessed with qigong and certain teachers amassed hundreds of thousands of followers. These teachers were known as the Grandmasters and were able to sell-out entire stadiums, where they would give qigong lectures to thousands of people for hours on end. Many of these styles of qigong produced what might be termed spontaneous release, when the practitioner feels an urge to move spontaneously, swaying and shaking, releasing *xieqi,* or pathogenic qi. There are many accounts of spontaneous healing in tandem with these events, and in general, it seems that this qigong fever had a hugely beneficial effect on the health of society. There were, in fact, more people practicing qigong than at any time in history—so much so that the demand for teachers produced a swath of new qigong styles and self-proclaimed masters.

As the qigong field developed in the late 1980s and early '90s, things got out of hand. This was at the same time when interest in qigong was rapidly expanding in the West. Not only was there a huge increase in charlatanism, similar to the situation in India, where miraculous claims abounded, but certain Grandmasters in China were becoming so popular that they formed a genuine threat to the monopoly of political power. One such teacher, Li Hongzi, announced himself as the new messiah and changed his qigong school into a religion, known as Falun Gong. The group protested against government oppression in 1998, which led to a nationwide crackdown on qigong and its practitioners. For several years, it was made illegal to publicly practice qigong in groups, and members of the Falun Gong cult were severely persecuted. In the mid-2000s the ban was lifted, but the nationwide fervor surrounding qigong has since diminished.

Because of this unusual history there has been a lot of misinformation in the transmission of qigong to the West, because what was already a complex cultural practice became convoluted during the qigong fever. However, something that is not often appreciated is that qigong, when practiced in an appropriate way, seems to have a huge potential for soothing trauma, both individually and socially. I believe one of the main reasons for the surge in popularity after the Cultural Revolution is that qigong has this healing ability, particularly when practiced in a social context. The process that underlies this power is also at play in Dien Chan facial reflexology. What we see in both these arts is a hidden dynamic between the two poles of the body, with one pole represented by the face and skull and the other by the belly and pelvis.

Before we explore the traditional understanding of this dynamic, let us look at the history and neurobiology of stress and trauma and recent scientific innovations in this field, for we will find a compelling parallel between the old and new.

. . . .

TWO

The Roots
of Stress & Trauma

There is a trinity of the brain, the body, and the
environment. That is, the brain, the body, and
the environment are intrinsically related. The brain
cannot exist without a (wider) body, the (wider) body
not without a brain, and the brain/body not without a
material and social environment. . . .

The term "trauma" does not and cannot pertain
to an event as such, because any event as an object is
co-constituted by, co-dependent on, and co-occurrent with
one or more experiencing and knowing individuals.

ELLERT NIJENHUIS

The concept of stress is relatively new. In common parlance it refers to
a mental-emotional distress that not only feels unpleasant but also has
negative physiological consequences. There is a lack of specificity when
using the word *stress* as it means different things to different people. It
can refer to a physiological stress to body tissues (like inflammation) or
a psychological stress to one's mind. This is regardless of whether one is

talking about anxiety, depression, shame, or grief. This ambiguity often hinders practical solutions to counteracting stress.

The term *stress* was adapted from the field of Physics in the 1930s by the Hungarian endocrinologist Hans Selye and only entered general public awareness in relation to health in the 1950s. Selye's research clearly linked stress to the development of many chronic diseases and poor health in general. There is now an agreed consensus that stress plays a key role in many chronic illnesses. What is less understood is how to de-stress and how to correctly advise people in decreasing stress. Everyone is quite unique in this regard as an activity that is blissfully relaxing and de-stressing for one person can be torment and agony for another. What this highlight is, is that stress is relative—its nature changes according to our personal relationship with it. The ambiguity and confusion surrounding the word *stress* stems from framing it as a fixed thing rather than a complex and relational process. Useful as the term is, this misunderstanding leads people toward the same interpretation of their bodies and minds as fixed things rather than fluid, changeable processes. This inevitably confounds attempts to ameliorate stress.

Methods of improving our relationship with stress are in actuality methods of improving our mind-body relationship. However, consciousness remains largely an enigma to science, with fierce debate surrounding what constitutes mind and what constitutes body. In the mainstream understanding there are many important unknown elements in the dynamic between the body and mind. Because of this, the concept of stress is potentially a way to avoid talking about how emotions and beliefs affect physical health, or to simply avoid talking about emotions at all, which is similar to the way in which placebo is referred to in a derogatory way, when in fact it clearly demonstrates the therapeutic power of consciousness and the healing potential of belief and emotion. Reframing our experience of stress and, more fundamentally, the relationship between mind and body, could significantly improve our health and well-being.

Whether or not we appreciate it, we have all been conditioned to think and behave as if our mind is somehow distinct from our body and that the physicality of the world is separate from the consciousness of the world. This conditioned understanding of separation is even implicit in the structure of our language and also leads to the tendency to frame the body and our sense of personhood as fixed and relatively unchanging objects. Being objective is a high virtue in our culture. The dark side of this virtue is that it increases our tendency to objectify one another, which is a hallmark of the rigid intolerance and fundamentalism that has sadly defined the cultural history of the past few hundred years. Once our relational subjectivity is stripped away it makes it much easier to strip away someone's personhood and humanity.

However, the very fact that we are conscious beings implies that a purely objective viewpoint is an impossibility. The scientific method depends on being as objective as possible so we can get the most truthful account of the world (or rather, the least false account). But if we take a clear-eyed view of ourselves, it becomes apparent that our feelings of well-being or stress are a distinct blend of physicality and consciousness. And so, the conundrum of consciousness is central to effectively addressing stress.

We are constantly changing, our cells are always fizzing with new life, and our personhood is ever new. Why is it then that we have such solid and unchanging ideas of ourselves? In a nutshell, it's a very useful survival mechanism to stake your place in the world. We have evolved to survive and to flourish, and forming an identity is a good first step toward survival. However, many such evolved instincts also delude us to the greater truths of the world. This delusion would have you believe that your body will stay the same, as well as your sense of self. Like an illusion of immortality, our whole culture clings to youth and shuns the uncertainties of illness and death. These are not hot topics, but coming to terms with the transience of our lives will bring the concept of stress into sharp focus. Just like ourselves, stress is not an objective thing, it is fluid and changes according to our particular stance and perspective.

Although the term *stress* alludes to a rupture in our understanding of body and mind, it is nevertheless a useful word to summarize when we are overwhelmed and held captive by our emotions. *Stress* can simply be a word that summarizes the negative effect of emotion and subjective feelings. Although we can link both emotions and stress to processes within our neurochemistry, brain, heart, and breath, the attempt to pinpoint an exact definition of stress is as futile as trying to pinpoint an exact correlation between emotions and brain circuitry.

When stress is framed as a fixed thing it is commonly oversimplified as being an entirely bad thing. This in turn frames being in fight-or-flight mode as unhealthy, as something that leads to adrenal fatigue and burnout. Useful as these metaphors are, stress cannot be simplified as a purely hormonal release of cortisol, and the phenomenon of burnout cannot be simplified as just an imbalance in our adrenaline levels. If this were so then just waking up in the morning would be considered stressful, or any demanding physical activity would be termed stressful. There are incredibly complex chains of interweaving psychobiological processes that interplay in the experience of stress. The nervous system, endocrine system, and cardiovascular system are all at the forefront of this, though there are many other influencing factors at play, including our childhood development, immune system, microbiome, and diet, as well as our genetic makeup and ancestral heritage, and even our social orientation and architectural environment. All these factors play a part in determining what type of relationship we have with stress.

There are aspects of stress that are positive and essential for living a healthy and fulfilled life. With gradual exposure to stressful situations, we become accustomed and normalized to them, which can develop our natural resilience.[1] What is key here is the word *gradual*. Time is a critical factor in our relationship with stress. When mildly stressful situations come in short bursts and have a defined finishing point, our bodies can then self-regulate and integrate our experience, which can have a very positive and stimulating effect on our health, immune system, and overall resiliency. A good example of this is the use of regular cold showers or cold-water swimming. When gradually brought into one's lifestyle these can have a positive effect on the immune system and general health, but if one were to simply jump into icy water without any preparation, the effect would be potentially life threatening. When we have a clear sense of the timeframe a stressful situation will last, this makes it much easier to withstand. But when stressful situations are drawn out over a long period of time and there is no endpoint in sight, our bodies and minds get overwhelmed and burned out, which can cause ill health.

As you can imagine, the complexity of life is such that we all have an array of stressful situations that are simultaneously playing themselves out over unknown time spans. The ability of the mind to create a space between what is happening now and what might happen in the future is an important skill in fashioning a truthful perception of our situation. As the great psychologist Viktor Frankl says, "Between stimulus and response there is a space. In that space is our power to choose our response. In our response lies our growth and our freedom."

Being mindful of the present moment is at the crux of a great majority of stress-management techniques. One reason for this is that the ability to finely focus our attention literally rewires our brain. So, when we can stay calm and present in each passing moment, even amid an unfolding crisis, this will re-pattern our brain and neurochemistry in real time so that our relationship with the crisis changes from being overwhelmingly stressful to simply challenging. As the saying goes, when it comes to the synaptic firing of brain activity, "what fires together wires together." This capacity to change our brain (and in fact our embodied experience) is called neuroplasticity. Although it tends to slow down after the age of twelve, research has shown that plasticity particularly occurs under three circumstances:

1. Shock—sudden and impactful experience
2. Novelty—new and interesting stimuli
3. Concentration—with the quality of paying close attention[2]

This is a both a saving grace and a double-edged sword, for negative thinking patterns also employ neuroplasticity. They can take up a lot of our attention, and so when a line of thinking becomes ingrained, it becomes much easier, and even addictive, to fall back on. The feeling of normalcy brings a sense of assurance and even comfort, even if it's associated with a line of thinking that's tinged with anxiety or anger. The mindfulness revolution has resulted in an explosion in the popularity of mindfulness techniques, but it is vitally lacking the nuance and context from which the word originates. Mindfulness is not a magic bullet, and in the case of people who have experienced violent trauma, mindfulness meditation has the potential to exacerbate symptoms of PTSD.[3]

The original Buddhist framework details specific actions that mindfulness plays in our consciousness. In the religious texts we have a clear description of right mindfulness and wrong mindfulness; hence, there was knowledge of the double-edged sword that mindfulness and neuroplasticity can represent. Right mindfulness rests on a foundation of virtue, which at its basis is the cultivation of self-restraint and non-violence in words, thoughts, and deeds. If a man is wholly fixated on killing someone, he can at the same time exemplify strong mindfulness and awareness of his intent. Even though he may develop strong mindfulness with his murderous intent, the end result won't lead to happiness or peace of mind—quite the opposite.

Unfortunately, some forms of trauma can leave such an imprint on the mind that they can undermine our attempts to establish right mindfulness. It is very important not to judge or blame, for when we or others feel broken by stress and trauma or for when mindfulness techniques are difficult to engage with, as it is more challenging and complex than is often realized. Again, what we are seeing is a mismatch of language and culture that belies a confusion about the nature of consciousness itself. Mindfulness is simple and at the same time infinitely complex.

Whereas in the West we assume that consciousness is bound within the brain and disconnected from everything outside of the skull, in the East consciousness has traditionally been understood as a process that unifies and connects the world. It is seen like an empty field in which everything and everyone is embedded. This naturally leads to framing ourselves and life as bound by relationship rather than through a lens of division and separation. The process philosophy of Alfred Whitehead echoes this intuition, that our mind and body fundamentally exist as processes—not as things. When we appreciate the ever-changing processional nature of self and world, this changes our values and places greater meaning on the relationship between two things rather than the things in and of themselves. As Wade Davis notes of the Penan Tribe of Borneo, "They measure wealth not by the extent of their possessions but by the strength of their relationships."[4]

This is a key factor when it comes to stress. We are by far the most social and communicative creatures on the planet. Unlike other mammals, we can work together in groups of millions, like ants or bees. This ultra-social nature has big benefits, as well as big disadvantages. Our sense of being bonded to others is a major factor in how we experience stress. When we are in the company of true friendships, we are more capable of handling stress. But when we have no friends and are completely isolated, then stress can be greatly magnified. Social isolation and loneliness have long been known to negatively affect our health and are a major compounding effect on stress, so the dynamics of our social lives play a pivotal role in our relationship with stress.

All societies are composed of vast networks, many of which are structured hierarchically. These hierarchies are constantly shifting and dictate the power dynamics in families, businesses, universities, hospitals, and all other forms of social organization. Research has shown that one's perceived place in a social hierarchy correlates with individual levels of cortisol, which is often taken as a rough marker for stress levels. The lower one is on the hierarchy, the greater stress one experiences.[5]

This might seem clear-cut, but the fact that we live our lives within multiple hierarchies introduces great complexity. We might be head of our family but at the bottom of one particular group of friends. We might be at the top position in business but in the lowest position in our family. This shows that our fundamental sense of status is the key to a healthy relationship with stress. It is important to note that our sense of status depends on particular sets of beliefs, assumed responsibilities, and the clarity of our self-perception. We all have the ability and freedom to change this. Research also shows that although the higher one is in a hierarchy, the less stress is apparent; this changes once one is at the top of the hierarchy, which is the most stressful place to be! The mentality of being happy only when one gets to the top is a disaster in waiting. If this attitude is tweaked, we can learn to live well and happily wherever we are in a social hierarchy. It is telling that the mediums for all social dynamics are the face, voice, and body language. By coming back to the face and body through touch and feeling we can begin to reorient both our sense of status and our relationship with stress.

In extreme cases, when a stressful experience overwhelms us, it has the potential to become traumatic. This can occur suddenly, such as in a traffic accident, or it can occur gradually, such as in the daily grind that eventually leads to a breakdown.

Both sudden trauma and slow or soft trauma can lead to a similar variety of symptoms. PTSD is also a relatively new concept, which was only recognized in the wake of the Vietnam War, when research with traumatized veterans and the convergence of different social advocacy groups prompted the official diagnosis. The actual experience of trauma is universal throughout human history—it is a basic and inevitable fact of living. But only recently have we developed greater insight into what is happening biologically both during and through the aftermath of trauma.[6]

Soldier's heart, Da Costa syndrome, railway spine, shell shock, battle fatigue, war neurosis, and combat stress reaction are all historical names for PTSD, and although it might sound like only soldiers suffer from it, this is only because soldiers go through such consistently traumatic experiences. In fact, anyone can suffer from trauma or PTSD. Aside from war veterans, the other group that has extremely high rates of trauma are people who have been abused in childhood, either emotionally, physically, or sexually. New understandings of trauma suggest that it is actually a hidden epidemic, for even if we haven't been abused as a child or in a war, there is a great, heaving undercurrent of trauma that plagues our history.

We are all, to a greater or lesser degree, being swayed by this undercurrent. As the great addiction specialist Gabor Maté says, "We live in a highly traumatized society," and the current crises we face in mental health and cultural meaning are both rooted in historical and personal trauma. We are all the walking wounded. For this reason, to address the most pressing health crisis of our times we need to frame it within the lens of stress and trauma—that is to say, within the prism of emotion, consciousness, and neurobiology.

One way to think of this is to see both stress and trauma as on a spectrum. At any given time, we have different levels of resiliency, which acts as our buffer against everyday stress or traumatic events. When our resilience is stretched to its limit, our bodies' adaptive intelligence finds ways to survive. But when the force of a stressful event exceeds our resilience, the stressful becomes the traumatic. Our natural survival instincts are forced into an extreme response, and sometimes our bodies struggle to come back to a natural balance after the event. The prevalence of developing PTSD or related symptoms after a traumatic event is higher than most people might assume but varies dependent on the current state and resilience of the person and the type and severity of the trauma.[7]

As mentioned before, the reasons why one person responds so differently to another is due to myriad factors that are unique to each person. It is important to understand that what is considered stressful is not proportional to each person's response. What can be good fun for one person can be a terrifying ordeal for another. Once we can step into another person's shoes and feel empathy, we can start to appreciate that there is a great subtlety and complexity to this dynamic.

There are two primary ways that the body reacts in extreme situations. When I say extreme, I mean situations that on some level feel life threatening and that we cannot talk our way out of or run away from. The first is to fight back and summon animal rage, which generally occurs in the presence of severe danger. However, if the danger is inescapable, life threatening, and we clearly have no chance in fighting, the other response is to physiologically shut down, which happens either by passing out or by feigning death. This playing dead jars our awareness from our body and releases the body's natural opioids, which are extremely potent painkillers. It is effectively a saving grace from having to fully experience the pain of dying a violent death. It is also a survival mechanism as predators have evolved to be wary of eating dead meat, and so playing dead creates the possibility of surviving such encounters. Sometimes flight, fight, and shutdown occur in sequence. Sometimes there is also a freeze response where we are highly aroused but physically immobilized. These various responses seem to utilize different aspects of our nervous system—they're not solely the domain of the sympathetic fight-or-flight nervous system.

After a traumatic event, a sense of safety needs to be established for the body to regain homeostasis. There are gradations of safety, but what is critical is for the breath and heart rate to return to a normal pattern, which is known as self-regulation. We have a natural ability to self-regulate, which is our ability to calm ourselves, soothe our body, and regain clarity of perception. Our natural capacity for self-regulation is the backbone of our resiliency. However, as a social species, our ability to self-regulate is greatly facilitated by the loving presence and assurance of another person. This co-regulation is particularly important for children and those with decreased capacity for self-regulation but helps us all. When we can reassure one another through our voice, facial expression, and presence, this begins the process of psychologically integrating the experience. It brings us back to homeostasis and a feeling of safety.[8] If this doesn't occur, we will hold the tension memory of the event throughout our mind-body, and symptoms such as flashbacks, panic, anxiety, nightmares, and dissociation might occur. As has been mentioned, a great many people experience these types of symptoms.

However, there is no consensus over what makes an event traumatic, which, like stress, results from the framing of trauma as a fixed thing rather than a relational process. There is actually very little clinical research into one of the key symptoms of PTSD, which is dissociation (to date there hasn't been one random control trial).[9] The subjective nature of dissociation is a big challenge for scientific research, akin to trying to study dreams or out-of-body experiences. In the general populace, research has shown that upward of 50 percent of people experience some form of transient/nonpathological dissociation, with estimates of up to 90 percent of people having experienced some form of trauma in their lives.[10]

In previous decades it was thought that PTSD was primarily a psychiatric disorder and, as such, its mechanism lay in the mind. The pioneering work of trauma specialist Bessel van der Kolk has demonstrated that the nervous system plays a fundamental role in trauma and PTSD. So much so, that within this framework PTSD could equally be called a dysregulation of the nervous system. This would classify PTSD as not only a psychiatric disorder but also akin to a physical injury, like suffering from a stroke.

The clinical psychologist Peter Levine further developed this line of thinking and developed a new way of understanding how all mammals and humans recover from trauma. By observing how mammals react and recover from predatory attacks in the wild, he realized that there was a universal process of discharging and releasing energy after surviving an attack. This takes the form of trembling or shaking, which assists the recovery and health of the animal. The same physiological process that supports survival for antelopes, deer, and mice is also supporting us humans. It's easy to understand this if you reflect on how a scary situation can make your hands tremble or how after an accident the whole body can tremble and shake. So rather than segregating PTSD as a disorder of the mind or even as an imbalance in the brain, Levine has shown that it is a whole-body phenomenon, in effect helping to shift our focus of healing from being purely in the head to being fully embodied. As the trauma therapist David Berceli succinctly states, "Healing trauma is about meeting the body."

Over the past few decades there has been a pioneering movement toward a more nuanced understanding of stress and trauma, catalyzed by innovative approaches at the intersection of psychotherapy, neuroscience, and evolutionary biology. Some of the most significant work has been made by Bessel van der Kolk, Peter Levine, Daniel Siegel, Stephen Porges, and Iain McGilchrist. Siegel has elucidated the phenomenon of neuroplasticity, showing that the brain has an incredible capacity to rewire itself and that mindfulness plays a key role in this, meaning that the biological underpinnings of who we are can change in radical ways and that we do not need to feel trapped by what has happened or who we have been in our past—we can change.

Porges has made groundbreaking work in the development of polyvagal theory, which shows us that the nervous system is much more complex and sensitive than once thought and that our social relationships are vital for health and healing. His work is of great significance because it shows that the sense of being safe is fundamental for health and healing. This has profound ramifications for all modern health care, for education and legal systems, for parenting, and particularly for the understanding of stress and trauma recovery.

McGilchrist has pioneered a new way of understanding the differences between the left and right brain hemispheres. His work shows that the two sides of the brain have distinct ways of paying attention and making sense of the world around us. The popular notion that the right brain is emotional and the left brain is logical is largely incorrect—both sides of the brain are involved in all the processes that were once thought to be one-sided. Emotion and cognition are interfused. In short, the two sides of the brain create different ways of attending to the world.

There are drastic implications if we only see the world primarily from the stance of one hemisphere or the other, and finding the right harmony between the hemispheres creates the most truthful attunement to the world around us. This refers directly back to whether we see ourselves and the world as mechanistic objects or as dynamic processes. McGilchrist's work is incredibly important for understanding both the crises that our culture faces and the close parallel between our self-perception and our perception of the world.

Just these three areas of research have the potential for a revolutionary shift, both on a global level and in our personal lives. However, these are only partial threads of a new and beautiful emerging vision of our biology and our spirituality. If we bring together older traditions of embodiment with this new avant-garde, we will see a significant and intriguing overlap.

Before we explore the older traditions there is a last, big factor that I would be remiss not to mention in this brief overview of stress and trauma. This is the role that both our early childhood and our family, cultural, and ancestral heritage plays in this relationship between stress and personhood.

When we first come into the world, we are in a state of extreme helplessness and vulnerability—our survival is entirely dependent on our caretakers. Physiologically, our brains and bodies grow and adapt to the world in an extraordinary way during these early years. This is fairly unique to humans. Our ability to self-regulate is actually outsourced to those around us, which includes not just our emotional equilibrium but also our thermoregulation. Our internal body sense and our social sense of self are both intimately shaped by these early years. A big part of this development is mediated by face-to-face interaction. We learn to feel safe and calm via the warmth of other faces and the soothing quality of other voices. Self-regulation is in fact bound up in co-regulation; in other words, our personhood is woven into the world around us.

From within the first hour of being born, we become fascinated with gazing at others' faces and begin mirroring facial expressions. Mimicry is fundamental to human culture. The capacity to connect with other human faces is actually instinctual, for it bonds us to those around us.[11] As helpless babies, this bond ensures that we are cared for and not abandoned. Beyond the darkness of reducing a baby's glance to an evolutionary survival strategy, what words and feelings could possibly describe the wonder we feel looking into a newborn's eyes? However we look at it, we are indeed molded and shaped by the faces and voices of those around us—it's a major part of who we are.

Intertwined in this early conditioning are the threat responses and subtle cues of stress and danger we pick up from those around us. We inherit the stress responses from our parents and caretakers. But the more we experience being held and supported by the safety net of our family, especially when graduating through the natural trials of growing up, the more resilience we will have. We will also enjoy better overall health and a more open capacity for nourishing relationships.

In the 1990s, a major research study came out that clearly linked the amount of stressful events through childhood with increased poor health and disease across multiple domains. Known as the Adverse Childhood Experience Study (ACES), the results unequivocally show that one's social environment as a baby and as a child has a tremendous effect on all aspects of adult health. There is a clear correlation between experiencing stressful events in one's childhood and a significantly increased likelihood of developing chronic and severe disease as an adult.

This adds a complex dimension to understanding trauma in adults. When people with difficult and stressful childhoods also experience traumatic events in later life, this layering of stress upon stress confounds any simple linear explanation of trauma. For this reason, many people are now diagnosed with complex PTSD (cPTSD), sometimes known as developmental trauma. There is also strong evidence that multiple personality disorder, currently known as dissociative identity disorder, is a form of cPTSD, having the same root causes in childhood development.[12]

As time goes on, there will probably be even further differentiation as the links between trauma and all types of disease are more firmly established. Intergenerational trauma has now been clearly documented, most notably in studies from holocaust survivors, but this can also be extended to many other communities, such as those suffering from the legacy of slavery and war. On the one hand, this is helpful if effective medication and treatment are discovered, but on the other hand, we risk missing the forest for the trees if our culture does not reframe how it fundamentally copes with, understands, and addresses trauma. As it stands, there is no effective medication for PTSD. There is also an incredible amount of disagreement as to the nature and definition of the diagnosis, with opposing camps in psychiatry, psychotherapy, and neurobiology.

Furthermore, over the past decade mainstream culture has started to become increasingly aware of the trauma-informed viewpoint. This is encouraging, but at the same time there is plenty of space for misunderstanding and oversimplification, such as seeing everything simply as childhood trauma, or labeling moderately annoying events, such as having a bad haircut or getting stuck in a traffic jam, as traumatic. The nuances of healing trauma and managing stress are missed when simplified into bite-size slogans. It can be reassuring to appear to have all the answers, and sometimes the pragmatic solution is to start with very simple baby steps, but the reality is that the cultural and historical roots of trauma lead us into complex and unknown terrain. It might just be that Rilke was right and that the full complexity of trauma should not be approached like it is a problem that can be fixed but rather as a mystery to be experienced. Approaching trauma as a thing that can be problem-solved might misrepresent the entangled reality of what trauma can be for some people. In other words, the mind-set we start out with may be a hindrance to fully grasping the scale and complexity of trauma.*

We cannot just treat the symptom and ignore the root. However, if we trace the roots back to their source, some difficult questions arise concerning our relationships and the relational patterns that run through our families, communities, and societies. How can we address the symptoms of this relational biology unless we go to the very heart of identity, culture, and society? As Nijenhuis states, "The realisation of childhood traumatisation requires societies to deeply reconsider exceedingly complex matters."[13] Our relationship with our self, mind, and body is a crucial dynamic in both stress and trauma. But how can we grasp this dynamic without a clear understanding of consciousness, the very thing that mediates our physical experience and well-being? What exactly is the relationship between consciousness and health?

The greatest minds of our scientific age have yet to find an answer to this hard question of how consciousness arises, let alone its supposed interaction with the pulsing of our heart or the growth of our bones. Modern doctors and therapists simply rely on the reductionist model

---

*For a deeper exploration into how our culture may be simplifying and commodifying the notion of trauma, I recommend the work of philosopher Bayo Akomolafe—particularly his dialogues with the poet and author Sophie Strand.

that the mind is entirely produced and contained in the brain, which is good so far as it goes but has some serious blind spots. There is no definitive evidence to show that the brain creates consciousness, and to date there is not even a viable scientific theory that can explain the jump from the firing of brain neurons to conscious awareness.[14]

It's simply an assumption to say that the partial correlation between aspects of the mind and the brain is proof that the brain causes consciousness. This is a low-resolution view of consciousness, reducing the full and wondrous complexity of consciousness to a bunch of synapses and brain neurochemistry. It works to a certain extent but also greatly limits our understanding of ourselves, our health, and nature at large. It seems that the scientific method itself lacks the ability to reconcile our dual subjectivity and objectivity, which lies at the very heart of consciousness. Because of this apparent paradox, many leading thinkers have sought to expand our framing of knowledge as more than being strictly objective or subjective, with nothing outside or in between. This is in keeping with the latest scientific evidence.

McGilchrist describes it this way: "We neither discover an objective reality nor invent a subjective reality, but there is a process of responsive evocation, the world *calling forth* something in me that in turn calls forth something in the world."[15] This mutual contingency is beautifully explained in the biologist Kriti Sharma's book *Interdependence,* which breaks down how this is actually occurring in the physiology of our sense perception. The physicist Carlo Rovelli also echoes this in his recent book *Helgoland,* describing how this relationality is occurring not just in our perception but also as a fundamental feature of reality. If we take these conclusions and bring them into our everyday lives, we'll see a strong parallel with the Buddhist doctrines of emptiness and interdependent origination. This way of seeing the world is most exquisitely described in the philosophy of Nagarjuna and in the little-known Chinese school of Hua Yan Buddhism. It's also paralleled by Western thinkers such as Wolfgang Goethe with his exact sensorial imagination and Henry Corbin with his Mundus Imaginalis. And so, we start to unthread a direct link between this way of approaching reality and the Dien Chan perception of seeing the entire person, or the entire world, within the face.

A useful word that helps us appreciate this new way of looking at ourselves was coined by the cognitive science professor John Vervaeke: the *transjective*. This describes a third way of knowing that is not entirely subjective nor purely objective. Instead, the transjective transcends this dualism and points toward a participation that takes place through our contact with reality, bringing us into closer contact with the truth and giving it a tangible quality in the here and now. Without the notion of the transjective, what is truthful can only be referred to in the highly abstract realm of scientific theory, which can lead to the hollowing out of our lived experience of the world, as if we are always one step removed from real life. This lends to the stereotype of the scientist as always being stuck in their head, stuck in abstraction.

By contrast, the transjective highlights our connectedness with life; it helps ground and embody our contact with reality. It also suggests that at a fundamental level we are participating in the creation of reality and are not merely temporary voyeurs of this world.

This should not be implied to say that we are the sole creators of our reality but rather that our consciousness and perception are dynamically coupled with the coming-into-being of the world around us. Although this might sound a little mystical, it can be framed as a natural part of our evolution. Our conscious perception is an active and co-creative force in the world. This has been proved again and again by physicists over the past seventy years. This is most readily known as the observer effect, made famous by the double-slit experiment.[16]

Many of the world's leading trauma therapists also find that working within a relational paradigm, meaning one that honors the patient's own experience and perceptions, proves to be the most effective. It's really just common sense—the way you look at someone changes the way they behave toward you. The way you look at the world interacts with its unfolding.

The transjective mode of being helps us gain access to truths that transcend the literal appearances of the world and integrate the symbolic dimensions of life, what the theologian David Bentley Hart calls "the dream language of myth and sacred art." This integration is essential if we are to approach the full import of trauma. A relational biology embraces not only the reductionist and the rational but also the imaginal and the more-than-human. This can then allow us to grapple with the crisis of meaning, as well as with morality, suffering, and death, areas that are so often entwined with trauma.

To be able to carry on living after experiencing tragedy is not something our modern medicine or culture is well equipped for. We often get stuck in a pretragic mode of thinking, preferring to stay in the naïveté of our idealism rather than confronting the crisis of our collective trauma and the cultural meaning crisis that is so prevalent in these modern times. Death is taboo, and the cyclical patterns of nature are fought against. When our mind-set is stuck in this pretragic mode we cannot mature into the fully polyrhythmic beings that we are. We can't access what's called post-traumatic growth.

Post-traumatic growth is often thought of as the reassembly of meaning and insight into life, which enriches our lives past what it was before the trauma. This kind of life experience might also be called wisdom. And in contrast to more linear forms of knowledge and meaning-making, wisdom accounts for the symbolic and polyrhythmic, the nonlinear and mythical dimensions of life. Wisdom dances with the immediacy of the unknown unknowns, that which is outside of our control, prediction, and even beyond human-centric ways of knowing.

Classical Chinese Medicine is a wisdom tradition—it engages symbolic language, and because of this it can penetrate past the singular meaning of things. It juggles multiple orders of truth at the same time.

As the sinologist Isabelle Robinet states, "The language of alchemy is a language that attempts to say the contradictory."[17] This only makes sense from a post-tragic mode of being, one that can hold in play opposing emotions and valid but competing statements of truth. A classic aphorism that describes this paradox is that "I don't want to suffer, but I greatly desire that which leads to suffering!"

Inside all of us there are competing evolutionary drives, or from a mythical perspective, we are composed of many characters who do not always get along. Long-term and short-term goals are a dry way of describing the fiendish entanglement between desire, yearning, and consequence. When we feel emotionally conflicted, the clarity of reason and logic are sometimes insufficient. This is when an alchemical language and way of seeing can give us space to see ourselves and each other from multiple perspectives. It is not simply ambiguous poetry, although by all appearances it may seem so. Rather, it's speech that's humbled by the sheer complexity and mystery of life, so much so that it dare not enclose meaning so tightly into literal definitions. *Yin, yang,* and *qi* cannot be literally defined and so are more closely aligned with the living nature of the world, which is always in a state of process and change. Because of this, complex situations can be transformed.

It is necessary to step beyond appearances if we are to grasp the role that consciousness plays in our bodies, and to do this requires coaxing our speech and language into unfamiliar terrain. Language forms the outer appearance of our thoughts, and so I implore you to look beyond the surface of these words and engage with your capacity for feeling, as it were, extending your heart's imaginative reach. Hart hints that this reaching out of the heart can precipitate a "sudden awareness that no mere fact can possibly be an adequate explanation of the mystery in which one finds oneself immersed in at every moment."[18] As later chapters will explore, this sense of awe and wonder plays a vital role in restoring our health and transforming old ways of thinking. That our consciousness is enmeshed with the world around us is truly wondrous.

Hart describes this sense of wonder as "an abiding amazement that lies just below the surface of conscious thought." Indeed, this is precisely what the Eastern traditions also point toward—an intimate and vivid interplay between the inner life and the world around us.

Therefore, we might gain fruitful insights if we explore some of these different traditions and ways of knowing. After all, for more than two millennia they have delved most deeply into the nature of the mind through contemplation and meditation. They also lie at the foundation of Dien Chan, qigong, and Classical Chinese Medicine.

Meditation should not be dismissed as a valid form of investigating the nature of consciousness, as it's entirely likely that our own mind is the only instrument we have at our disposal that is powerful enough to reveal the truth about consciousness. Of course, we retain the value of shifting back into more scientific modes of discovery, where we have safeguards in place against bias and cognitive dissonance. The precision of empiricism and specificity of reason are vital tools. But these tools are not universal keys that can unlock all mystery. The bare fact doesn't reflect the deep truth. Data must always be interpreted through the prism of our human limitations. This is where I hope that the modern science of trauma and the old traditions of healing can come into dialogue, in this liminal space between indigenous and modern vantage points.

There are incredible healing tools that can be learned from both the modern and ancient paradigms. What's often hidden in our modern search for healing trauma is the interconnection between the personal, social, and ecological. Our modern culture is hyperindividualistic. Therefore, special mention is made in later chapters of not just the self-care techniques we can learn for self-healing but also the relational and communal healing practices such as the Shen Ren Dao system of virtue healing from northern China and the Ho'oponopono system of Hawaii, both of which gift us with beautiful ways of healing trauma and emotional conflict within our families and communities.

One of our major cultural limitations that inhibits us from fully appreciating indigenous ways of knowing and healing is the conviction that the brain is the sole domain of consciousness. This conviction, while seemingly rational and anti-magic, strips away awe and mystery from life. But for all we think we know, consciousness is indeed still a mystery to us. Let us be willing to be open to possibility.

In the Eastern traditions there are different notions of what is possible when it comes to the mind. There is a recognition that consciousness occurs throughout our body. Our face, eyes, heart, and belly are creative aspects of our conscious experience—it's not just confined to the brain. By exploring the energetic dynamic between the head, face, and body, we will come to learn about the different modes of consciousness that arise from different ways of embodiment. Understanding the polarity that lies between our head and body creates the foundation for understanding Dien Chan and the universal process that it harnesses.

. . . .

THREE

The Energetic Dynamic between the Face & Body

Learn the backward step that turns your light inward
To illuminate within.
Body and mind of themselves
Will drop away
And your original face will be manifest.

DOGEN

Why do we have a face? What is the original purpose of our face, head, or brain? Such a simple and seemingly obvious question, but we will see that it pulls on a thread that is entangled in great unknowns.

Our face exists to bring energy into our body. This is an evolutionary answer. To be alive requires a constant stream of air flowing through our faces. Our mouth, teeth, and jaw energize us through the ingestion of water and food. Our eyes and ears evolved to optimize our intake of air, food, and water. Then, through the evolutionary process of exaptation, we discovered that this mouth and breath of ours can also be repurposed for speech. Our faces found language. And what would we be without the richness of our storied tongue?

The expressivity of the face also displays our intentions, emotions, and nonverbal communications, which is especially important for us as a hypersocial species. We've evolved to use our faces instinctively to cue one another to potential threats, thereby enhancing our collective survival. Furthermore, because our faces are the primary way in which we recognize one another, this part of our body is particularly bound up in notions of self-identity and status. Our faces both attune to and regulate the bodies of those around us while at the same time being enmeshed with our own brain and helping to regulate our own body state.

Our brains evolved, like other animals, to help regulate our bodies. Our brains are in service to our bodies. Just like our tongue and teeth were co-opted for creating language, our brains have also moved toward complex thinking, reason, story, and abstraction. Because of this, our culture has come to think of our brain as the seat of intelligence and our thinking organ. We tend to forget its role as the administrator for the body. It is because of our cultural bias that we tend to deny the intelligence of our body, to deny that our heart and abdomen might have something intelligent to contribute.

We also tend to oversimplify the complex relationship between thoughts and feelings, assuming that our cognition is somehow disconnected from the body as a whole. Many people now assume our brain is the container of both our personhood and consciousness itself and believe that we could transfer our identities to another body purely via brain transplant or escape the body entirely by uploading our neural makeup to the internet. This kind of thinking is reflective of a wider cultural trend that places the head and the brain as superior and special and somehow disconnected from the rest of our body. By contrast, the body is relegated to something that has evolved merely to carry the head around.

In the same vein, the mind is understood to be located in the skull and consciousness then somehow conjured up within our brain tissue. Much of this thinking has roots in the ancient Greek philosophy that lies at the foundation of Western culture, but there is also a strong component that comes from the Judeo-Christian conception of body and soul. It runs deep and posits that everything above is divine and everything below is hell. Our head is closest to heaven and is blessed with divine reason. Our body is mired in the muck of the Earth and is framed as a brutish animal. How do we step back from this simplistic but deeply held conditioning?

Let's imagine what our face and mind might've seemed like to someone outside of this perspective. In ancient China and Japan, for instance, the umbilicus and lower abdomen were taken as the central component of our being, both geographically and metaphysically. Known as the Hara in Japan and as the Dan Tien in China, these parts of our body were considered the root source of our life, the reservoir of potential and core foundation of both mind and body.

In classical Buddhism, Daoism, and Chinese medicine, the mind is not understood to be a product of the brain but rather a process of the heart. In many cultures the chest and belly are equally as important as the head and brain when considering where mind and identity truly reside. But this is of course an oversimplification that betrays the greater context of how life and consciousness were framed within the old traditions of China and East Asia.

In simple terms, the mind and matter that make up a human being parallel a greater pattern of consciousness and materiality within nature. This pattern is characterized not by a mind-body duality but by a trinity. The three components of this trinity are called yin, yang, and qi, the mediating factor between them.

Yin can be described as the movement toward materiality, and yang toward mentality. Qi is the pivot and enabling principle behind all movement and change in the world. The nature of this pattern of trinity is one of continuous change and transformation. As such, qi in the broadest sense could be defined simply as *change*. Yin and yang support and balance one another yet also transform into one another. They are not separate but always relative. This is how the ancient Chinese related mind to body, too—not as divided things but rather with each as part of a process of ever-changing relationship and transformation.

The seed of this way of understanding the body and world comes from the Yi Jing, or Book of Changes. Like a tree, the whole of Chinese culture branched out of this foundational tome. It informs the framework behind both Dien Chan and Chinese medicine.[1] It is also a famously obscure text that lends itself to multiple interpretations. From out of the Yi Jing, we can infer a unique way of approaching life, one that at its heart hinges upon resonance, change, and relationship. This is the language the concepts of yin, yang, and qi describe.

The dynamic between our head and body is a prime example of yin and yang. At the crown of our head there is an acupuncture point called Hundred Meetings (Du 20/*Bai Hui*). This point is considered the most yang aspect of our body. All the pathways of qi converge here in a unique way. Likewise, all the yang channels of the body either initiate or culminate on the face around the eyes, ears, nose, or mouth. This reflects the nature of yang, which is emblematic of action, fire, uprising, and manifestation. At the opposite end of our body, at the base of our pelvis, is the most yin point, known poetically as Seabed (Ren1/*Hui Yin*). The nature of yin is of nonaction, water, and gestation. By extension, the head and the abdomen form a dynamic between the yang and yin aspects of our embodiment. They form a bipolarity, held together by our centerline, our own personal axis mundi.

When we shift our attention and awareness along this central axis (see figure 3.1), we also shift our relationship with our body. Although this may at first seem like a small change in our attention, by actively feeling down through the body we can change both our physiology and, in a fascinating way, our mental state and perception. This can best be described as shifting between different modes of being.

For example, notice how you feel if you drop all your attention into

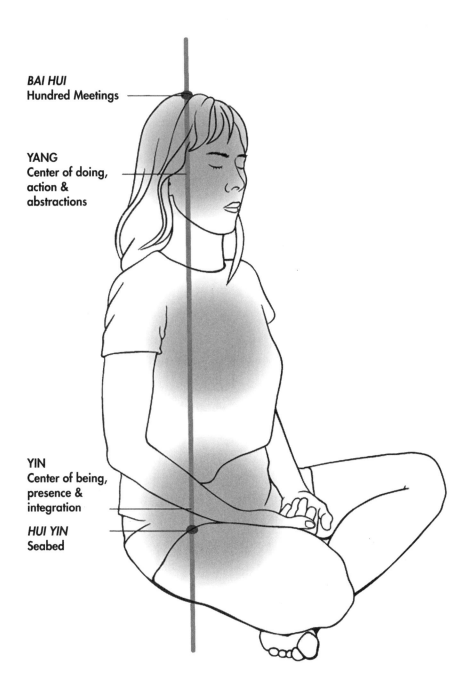

BAI HUI
Hundred Meetings

YANG
Center of doing,
action &
abstractions

YIN
Center of being,
presence &
integration

HUI YIN
Seabed

Figure 3.1. The energetic dynamic between the face and body

your chest—really feel it. Then feel farther down and try to rest your awareness within your abdomen. Did you notice your heartbeat? Our ability to feel down into the body like this is both completely natural and at the same time something that can be disconnected from. We can lose touch with the felt sense of our bodies.

Similar to the way we all have different postural habits and ways of holding our bodies, we also have different habits of body awareness. For some people, resting inside the body feels unpleasant, and so they disconnect from their feeling capacity. This can happen in many ways, either by becoming numb or holding our awareness above the neck, on the surface of the body, or even just outside of the body. This happens particularly alongside issues of chronic pain, trauma, and stress. Often the word *dissociation* is used to describe this numbing of our felt sense of the body.

However, this phenomenon is not unique to people with trauma—we all have different degrees to which we can feel inside various parts of our bodies; we all have shadow parts we rarely, if ever, feel in to. Just lightly feeling down into our body, we might get the impression that it's an inconsequential thing that has little bearing on our health. Yet there are great degrees to how deeply we can listen into our bodies, and this has a direct effect not only on our health but on all aspects of our lives as well. Our habits of embodiment play a significant role in health and healing. There is so much complexity and nuance in each person's way of inhabiting their body. This isn't only a matter of the person's individual history but also the family, the culture, and even the architectural and societal environment they grew up in.

In qigong, which reflects the general approach to embodiment from ancient Chinese culture, the first principle is to sink the qi. Sometimes this is called emptying the heart and filling the belly. Essentially it involves bringing our awareness down from the head and into the body. This trajectory, from the yang center of our body to the yin center, parallels several life processes.

The most obvious is the gastrointestinal tract—we take in food and water through our mouths, which then pass downward through our body. Interestingly, this process of digestion occurs not only with food but also with emotion, thought, perception, and experience. We seem to take in the world through the face, eyes, and ears—absorbing the world around us.

However, we can only digest and integrate these experiences and emotions if we let them flow through us, down into our core. If we stay up in our heads, we may register what is happening, but we don't fully absorb the experience. From this understanding, the mental space of our pelvic bowl and abdominal cavity allows us to dwell within our experience and be fully present to others.

Inhabiting this space can also bring us in touch with all the past experiences that remain undigested or unintegrated. The lower abdomen is the center of our being, a golden key to unlocking our capacity to deeply relax the mind and become emotionally balanced. By contrast, our head affords us the capacity to stand apart, separate our self, and draw perspective on the world. The head is the center of action and abstraction.[2]

As I mentioned before, the culture we are born into influences our habits of embodiment. Our parents teach us how to regulate our bodies, because as infants we cannot self-regulate. As we grow up we learn how to relate to our bodies and emotions by copying and being taught by our parents and teachers, who are in turn conditioned through our culture. Western culture as a whole has gradually, over the centuries, become more and more head centric and less connected to the subtleties of the felt body. The proclivity for abstraction, critical thinking, and reason has had incredible benefits. However, there is a downside. Even our language, which considers downward as bad, shows that this phenomenon needs some cunning if we are to properly frame it.

The problem with living only from our heads is that we lose touch with everything. When this becomes extreme, we lose the ability to relate to others, we become fixed into a type of narcissism and fundamentalism causes us to see the world from only one vantage point. As the historian Yuval Harari has noted, "Fundamentalism is becoming a defining trend of modern peoples."

Nevertheless, it would be a mistake to assume that this phenomenon of being stuck in our heads is purely a Western feature. It's actually a universal tendency, because there is also a biological basis for this bias of the head over the body. Having all our energy shoot up to the head activates our survival mode—we open our eyes and ears wide to alert ourselves to incoming threats. Conversely, resting our energy in the core of our body opens us to different ways of seeing. It brings us toward the world rather than buffering us from it and places us within a relational mode of being that is open to being changed by the world, that is in dialogue with the flux and flow that is always occurring between our body and everything around us. Different cultures grapple and respond to this dynamic in different ways. The process of "emptying the heart and filling the belly" is the Daoist response to this tendency.

In qigong culture there is also the prerogative "Bu Sheng Qi, Bu Shang Huo," which translates as "do not raise qi, do not flare up fire" and refers to the physiological effect of emotions and the detrimental effect that certain feelings have when they surge upward into the head. This ability to direct our awareness downward into the body I refer to as the *downward flow*. This flow parallels another important anatomical pathway, the vagus nerve, which originates in the cranium and descends from the face down through all the organs of the body, resting in the Seabed of the pelvic floor. The vagus nerve allows us to feel all the internal sensations of the body. This is called interoception, and it not only informs our brains of what is happening in our heart or liver but also is largely responsible for giving us the felt sensation of having a body. We will explore the relationship between Dien Chan, qigong, and the vagus nerve in the next chapter, for this forms a crucial link between ancient wisdom and modern understanding.

The energetic dynamic between our face and our body is one of continual change and transformation. To live well and be healthy we must be able to adapt to our world, which is also constantly changing. This requires us to be able to shift between these different modes of being that are activated by inhabiting the three cavities of our body—the cranium, the thorax, and the abdomen. It is common knowledge that our chest and heart bring us in touch with the emotions of life, and our gut and belly connect us to the intuitive and erotic. What is less commonly known is that increasing our ability to shift between these different centers has incredible health benefits and implications for our lives as a whole. When we come down into our center, we actually strengthen our vagus nerve, increasing what is called vagal tone. This not only enhances our ability to digest and integrate the world, but it strengthens our capacity for intuition, emotional intelligence, and eros as well.

Being fully embodied increases our balance, both physically and energetically. A balanced life must include a sense of intuition, emotional clarity, and eros. Embodiment allows us to approach the wholeness in life, and this occurs by opening to the full experience of our whole body. Like I mentioned before, most people have long-held habits of embodiment and tend to have diminished spots of body awareness, such as in the lower back or shoulder blades. It is actually quite rare to be fully aware, with crystal clarity, of our whole body as a unified experience. When we focus on using our hands or communicating with our face, there is often a tendency to forget what's happening in our feet or belly. Given the benefits of vagal tone and being in touch with our bodies, what is the natural way to increase and maintain our embodiment?

The natural way to find balance is to return to our center. When we align our center of awareness with our center of gravity this spreads our awareness equally through the whole body.* This whole-body awareness in turn has several effects. It helps decompress and decontract physical and emotional tension, allowing for a sense of spaciousness, flow, and release. It also shifts us toward what I call our holographic self. We become aware of how we are embedded within time and space, not as an isolated unit passing untouched through the world but instead as embedded through our connectivity and relationality.

This shift from embodiment to embeddedment opens us to the greater wholes that we are part of, both within our immediate geography and within what the Indigenous Australian people call Dreamtime. Instead of seeing life as a mechanical linear sequence of events, the holographic self resonates through a vastly interconnected web, like fractal geometry in all directions of space-time. When we return to our center, this activates a resonance that carries us toward healing and growth. This notion is the underlying principle behind Dien Chan and Chinese medicine. Therefore, the term Zhong, which translates variously as "center," "middle," "upright," or "heart," holds center stage in Chinese medicine. We will return to this theme in later chapters.

The practice of Dien Chan, both as a therapy and through self-care massage, utilizes the holographic principle that is at play within our mind-body. Coming into a felt relationship with this principle will slowly enhance our potential for the healing power of Dien Chan, which in actuality is the innate healing power of our mind-body. It can also open us to spiritual dimensions that lie just beyond the threshold of normal perception.

The initial step toward both healing and transformation is not forward or upward but down and back. In Zen meditation this is called the backward step and involves literally shifting back from the surface

---

*The alignment of our physical and mental posture is a key component of qigong, but I believe the most advanced postural teachings are most readily accessed through tai chi chuan. I am indebted to the incredible teachings of Sifu Yeung Ma Lee and her advanced student Murray Douglas for my understanding of this alignment.

of the face, allowing the release, and letting go of all masks, discovering our *original face*.[3] Dien Chan helps release the tension and holding patterns in the face, head, and neck, which in turn helps open all the energetic pathways between the head and body, allowing us to more easily settle and rest our awareness into the chest and abdomen. Dien Chan reconnects our head to our body, opening the downward flow into our vagus nerve and embodiment. This downward flow and the internal alchemy between the different spaces of our body is known in the qigong traditions as Jin Dan, the cultivation of the Golden Elixir. It's fascinating to realize the many parallels between Golden Elixir practices, Dien Chan, and the modern discoveries surrounding stress, trauma, and the vagus nerve.

FOUR

. . . .

The Golden Elixir
& the Vagus Nerve

The imagination is a powerful solvent—it keeps things fluid and prevents the world from freezing up. It breaks down walls. It refuses the literal and sees all things as metaphoric and symbolic.

TOM CHEETHAM

If we consider the spectrum of practices that fall under the umbrella term of qigong, the practice of the Golden Elixir is on the far side of the meditative and spiritual end. In Chinese culture, the Golden Elixir is deeply embedded within mythology and storytelling and could also be seen as a pinnacle of Daoist religious practice. The Daoist adept Liu Yiming described it as follows:

Golden Elixir is another name for one's fundamental nature, formed out of primeval inchoateness (Hun Cheng, a term derived from the Dao De Jing). There is no other Golden Elixir outside one's fundamental nature. Every human being has this Golden Elixir complete in himself: it is entirely realized in everybody. It is neither more in a sage, nor less in an ordinary person. It is the seed of Immortals and Buddhas, and the root of worthies and sages.[1]

This description gives us the impression that the Golden Elixir is at once both commonplace and sublime. It is a core feature within all of us, and yet its renown points to a near magical ability for self-healing and longevity, among other things.

From outside appearances, it involves meditation, breathwork, and visualization combined with body conditioning and self-massage. Beyond appearances, it's approached as an alchemical task. The type of alchemy here is different from the kind epitomized by the medieval Western pursuit of the philosopher's stone; rather, it's known as internal alchemy, and it seeks to transmute the base elements in our own consciousness and physicality to bring about a transformation of the world. This transformation is symbolically called Jin Dan (Golden Elixir) but is also referred to as Golden Flower, Golden Pill, or Inner Skill. It's closely associated with the mountain hermit tradition and the symbolic or literal pursuit of immortality.*

There is a close connection between the Golden Elixir practice and the healing traditions of China, as they share in the belief that the human body has an innate capacity for self-healing. The practice of the Golden Elixir is a catalyst for both physical health and spiritual evolution; the domains of medicine and spirituality traverse each other. And so many of the greatest physicians in history were also adepts of the Golden Elixir and were considered not simply as doctors but also as wise sages. Legendary historical doctors such as Ge Hong and Sun Si Miao owe their stature not only to book knowledge or clinical experience

---

*The Chinese character for *immortal* is Xian and can refer to a person attaining great physical longevity, with many accounts of adepts living well over one hundred years and even two hundred years. It also refers to spiritual immortality in the sense of creating a spiritual body that carries on after death and can also can refer to physical immortality in the literal sense, which would be a useful attribute for any martial artist.

but also to the direct insight gained through their inner exploration of these meditative practices.

The Golden Elixir practice has a direct overlap with Dien Chan facial reflexology. Many of the self-massage techniques of the Golden Elixir practice are the same as the self-care practices of Dien Chan. Although this isn't overtly talked about or demonstrated in Vietnam, this similarity suggests a hidden mystical dimension to Dien Chan. This is a running theme in many of the traditional arts of the East— the existence of a subtle bridge between the most mundane everyday activity and the most profound and sacred. Tea drinking is a perfect example.

However, if we cross-reference these types of massage techniques with the physiological underpinnings that inform the modern understanding of healing trauma, we'll see there's also considerable resonance.

There are essentially two factors that are striking. The first is the healing dynamic of the vagus nerve, which connects our face to our heart and our belly. The second is the social orientation network that aligns both our sense perception and our emotional regulation. Both Dien Chan and the Golden Elixir work with the energetic dynamics that exist between the face, the heart, and the abdomen and so undoubtedly engage the vagus nerve. They also create shifts in both our internal perception of the body, our emotional balance, and our external perception of the world.

What follows is my own speculation as to how these intriguing connections between ancient Eastern healing meditation practices and modern Western neuroscience show us maps toward healing and personal evolution.

The importance of the vagus nerve for our general health and healing cannot be overemphasized. The vagus nerve is known as the wandering nerve, for it is like a vagabond who that wanders through all aspects of the body. It is a cranial nerve, emerging from the brain stem behind the ear, and travels through the face and throat, down into the heart and lungs, and through the diaphragm into nearly all the organs of the belly. It forms the parasympathetic branch of our autonomic nervous system (ANS), the side responsible for our rest-and-digest mode. Because of this, it is sometimes called the antianxiety nerve as it acts as a counterbalance to the parasympathetic branch of the ANS, which is our fight-or-flight mode.

It also enables the tend-and-befriend response to stress, as the vagus nerve forms a key part of our social orientation network. The vagus nerve ties together our social communication, threat detection, and our internal regulation. Its pathway intimately connects our facial expression, hearing, and voice with the nerves that regulate the heart and breath.

Stephen Porges's polyvagal theory explains how the vagus nerve specifically mediates different aspects of our social orientation network. He shows how the vagus nerve contains two anatomically distinct branches, which he postulates have different functions. The frontal vagus branch (often called the ventral branch) innervates the face, heart, and lungs. This branch is formed of myelinated nerves, which means they are superconductive, just like in the brain. This enables the nuances and real-time complexity of our social orientation mode. The lower vagus branch (often called the dorsal branch) descends into the abdomen and pelvis and is unmyelinated. This lower branch is thought to be connected with our shutdown mode, which causes people to faint and dissociate under life-threatening circumstances. It is also connected with what Porges calls "immobilization with safety," which allows our bodies to come into close physical intimacy. If we pair these two branches of the vagus nerve alongside our fight-or-flight response from the parasympathetic nervous system, this means that instead of our ANS being a seesaw between sympathetic and parasympathetic, it can then actually be seen to have three different aspects. When these aspects interact with one another

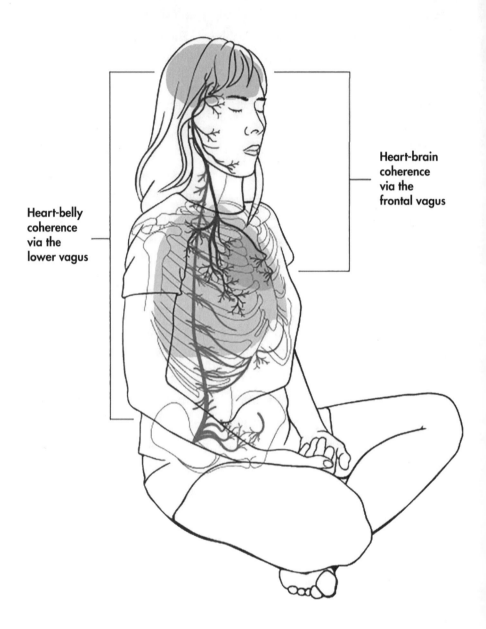

Heart-belly coherence via the lower vagus

Heart-brain coherence via the frontal vagus

Figure 4.1. Artist's rendition of the vagus nerve detailing the ventral and dorsal

they create five distinct modes that enable our complex human behavior:

- fight/flight
- rest/digest
- freeze/fawn
- play
- intimacy

For instance, when our social nervous system (our frontal vagus) is engaged but we are in violent competitive sports like rugby, this enables us to be in a playful mode and refrain from taking the rough and tumble as a personal threat to our lives. When both branches of our vagus nerve are engaged, this can enable intimacy, to immobilize with safety. This means that we can safely release ourselves into the close physical embrace of lovers, massage and therapy involving touch, or breastfeeding.[2]

When the vagus nerve is functioning well, we say there's strong vagal tone, which reflects our capacity to stay calm and socially engaged. Strong vagal tone is also associated with healthy heart and liver function, optimal breathing, a balanced microbiome, sleeping, digestion, and heightening our capacity for interoception, which gives us our felt sense of having a body.

There is compelling evidence that interoception plays a key role in maintaining our concept of self and is therefore foundational to mental health.[3] The researchers who investigated this suggest that increasing the capacity for interoception might be the key to solving many psychiatric disorders in which the concept of self is fragmented or unstable. The vagus nerve also plays a major role in reducing inflammation.[4] Too much inflammation in the body is a hallmark of our modern age and a significant underlying cause of a large percentage of modern diseases. The vagus nerve is crucial to living healthily, and contrary to what was previously thought, we have the power to influence and increase our vagal tone.

This means that we can increase our overall mental and physical health in ways that science had previously thought impossible. Therefore, the autonomic nervous system was first named autonomic, as it automatically keeps the heart beating and all the functions of our organs working with zero conscious input. Thank goodness it's all taken care of, and we don't have to micromanage our liver enzymes and heartbeat! However, it is now known that we can positively influence the vagus nerve and thereby affect the ANS. We can influence the ANS most directly through our breath, which is both autonomic and possible to consciously control. This is because we have evolved both on land and in water, and to effectively swim without drowning we need to be able to hold and have nuanced control over our breath.

Coincidentally, the so-called diving reflex, which happens anytime the face is submerged in water, is a wonderful way to stimulate the vagus nerve. This happens when swimming but can be triggered easily by splashing cold water onto your face one to three times. Branches of the vagus nerve innervate both the diaphragm and our lungs, and so learning to optimize our breathing (an important part of qigong and yoga) can strengthen our vagal tone. We can also influence the vagus nerve through both physical touch and the touch of awareness, a hidden benefit of both massage and meditation.

By touching our face, throat, chest, and belly, we can come into a felt experience of the vagus nerve. These areas of the body are unique in that they're often highly charged with emotion. If a stranger comes and puts his hand on your face or your chest or belly it will surely illicit a strong emotional response, and one that is quite different from had he placed his hand on your arm or back. This is because these parts of our body are the most vulnerable. The face, throat, and chest also play a pivotal role in the social nervous system—our social orientation mode. The frontal branch of the vagus nerve, which forms a key part of this system, connects the expressivity of our face and the intonation of our voice with the intelligence of our heart. The sense organs and how they light up our experience of the world also play a key role. A considerable proportion of our brain activity is taken up by the creation of our sense perception. In particular, our vision takes up more than 30 percent of measurable brain activity. Our vision, hearing, smell, and sense of other people instinctively and continuously scan for cues of danger or safety. This in turn cues whether we remain alert and on guard or relaxed, socially engaged, and attuned to healing.

When it comes to stress and trauma, the vagus nerve is identified as an essential component in healing and psychological recovery because the vagus enables our relationality, and both stress and trauma are relational by nature.

Each person's stress response is unique, which explains why two soldiers who go through the exact same situation can be affected in completely different ways—this is the relational nature of our mind and physiology at work. Dien Chan releases points of physical and emotional tension in the face, which in turn releases a cascade effect through our vagus nerve and social orientation network. It activates the sense portals of the body, which can re-pattern our sensorial apprehension of the world. I believe that this is a part of the reason why Dien Chan was so effective and popular in the aftermath of the Vietnam War—it was tapping in to the vagus nerve's ability to soothe and heal the trauma of war. However, I do not believe that its healing power can be entirely reduced to the workings of the vagus nerve, as the holographic principle (ganying) that is at play in both acupuncture and reflexology has a deeper power.

The Golden Elixir practice uses self-massage techniques that are by appearance the same as Dien Chan. By massaging the face, the intention is to open the energetic pathways that converge in the head, thereby increasing our clarity of perception and cognition. This is known as allowing the clear yang to rise. However, the Golden Elixir practice is of a different nature from Dien Chan. It has a two-thousand-year heritage, whereas Dien Chan has only been in existence for some forty years. In my understanding, Dien Chan can be placed within the overarching and complex heritage that finds its source in the Golden Elixir.

It would be a mistake to talk of the Golden Elixir from a strictly third-person narrative, as the reality is that there are many variations of the practice. I'm not a scholar of the Golden Elixir, and my understanding relies substantially on my personal practice and what wisdom I have gleaned from my teachers.* However, the different variations of the practice share some key features, one of which is that it is spoken of in symbolic language. This twilight language has the function of maintaining secrecy and keeping direct person-to-person transmission, which is done for protection of both the lineage and for students who might not be suited to or even harmed by the practice. More than this, symbolic language conveys beyond the literal, pointing toward a multi-dimensionality of being.

Rather than being straightforward, engaging with the Golden Elixir brings a person into a nonlinear experience of reality, something that is generally beyond our normal capacity for words. As the somatic historian Scott Park Phillips explains, "Golden Elixir practices are endless

---

*There are different branches of Daoism that hold their own versions of the Golden Elixir, and there are non-Daoist lineages connected to martial artists and scholar-doctors. Some lineages are modern, some are ancient or extinct. My personal practice comes from the American teacher Michael Lomax, who in turn learned it from Wang Juemin. Wang Juemin transmitted these teachings from some of the most famous qigong practitioners of the twentieth century, including Hu Yao Zhen and Chen Yingning. For more information on the resurgence of this lay branch or scholar branch of Jin Dan, see Xun Liu, *Daoist Modern: Innovation, Lay Practice, and the Community of Inner Alchemy in Republican Shanghai* (Cambridge Mass.: Harvard University Press, 2009). The more commonly taught practices come from the Dragon Gate Lineage, as taught by masters like Wang Liping or in the West, Damo Mitchell. There are also many very different styles of practice that stem from Mao Shan Daoism, which are found throughout Southeast Asia and in the overseas Chinese community.

loops, cycles, beginning in emptiness, taking form, and then returning to emptiness. They are processions of spatial order and simultaneous action."[5] Given this, any linear description is always just one side of a multifaceted prism. Like trying to keep hold of a frantic wet fish, the harder we grasp at understanding the interpenetration of form and emptiness, the easier it slips by us.

Again, this resonates with the overlapping nature of the commonplace and the sublime. Whereas the "normal" understanding of this might be that it involves some strange mechanism in the brain, there is a hint here that the vagus nerve may be potentially involved in heretofore unknown aspects of consciousness.

One aspect of the Golden Elixir is that it strongly establishes a felt sense of the body and the different potentialities that arise between our conscious and physical experience. Another way of describing this is that the Golden Elixir engages the nexus between our imagination, body, and perception. Instead of thinking of the imagination as pure fantasy, as in "it's just your imagination," we should give more recognition to the nuanced interaction between our minds and the construction of our reality. Considering the way that our attention, beliefs, and emotions change our sensuality and interpretation of the world, we might reframe the imagination as an organ of perception. Neuroscientists call this predictive processing, but it harkens back to a famous Talmudic adage—we see the things not as they are, we see things as we are. The imagination is especially pertinent to the vagus nerve, for our internal body perception and self-regard is anything but objective. As the scholar Tom Cheetham tells us: "There is a tight complementarity between emotions and the imagination."[6] And as we'll explore in later chapters, emotion is deeply woven into our interoception, which is mediated through our vagus nerve. It may be useful to adopt the term *imaginal* to refer to this creative aspect of being that is at once nonliteral and at the same time rooted in our physiology.

It's worth noting here that our own understanding of our body is most usually heavily informed by medical science and less so by direct personal experience. We rely on an anatomized body when we discuss what's happening inside us, and this is largely disconnected from the felt body. For example, who really knows where the spleen is? Can we spatially pinpoint the spleen within our body? And if we happen to have this knowledge, it most certainly comes from an anatomy textbook rather than from our personal experience, and so we are overlaying our own ideas and understanding over the direct felt sense of the body. The great benefits of having a detailed knowledge of anatomy are not in dispute. The problem lies in how our medical knowledge changes our cultural and personal perception of our own bodies.

The historian Ivan Illich has documented that this shift away from being in touch with our felt body occurred in Europe about one thousand years ago, when philosophy and medicine were separated from each other. This happened in part due to the establishment of the first European universities and hospitals. He says, "Philosophy was deprived of the body, and the body was deprived of its cosmic belonging."[7] In China, philosophy has traditionally been the bedrock of medicine. This of course has its own problems, but a great advantage is that it significantly opens up different ways of engaging with our physicality, ways that are exploited in the Golden Elixir. For an interesting glimpse into the symbolic realms of our body, look at the *Neijing Tu,* a painting that maps the mythical process of the Golden Elixir. Although we are speaking of the same body, the anatomized body reduces it to a collection of mechanical parts and in extremis can miss the contingent relationships between each part, leading to a sense of being disconnected, whereas the felt body connects all aspects of our mind-body into a resonant web of relation and interconnection.

Nevertheless, there are of course natural parallels between the anatomized body and the felt body. An important parallel is seen in the three cavities of our body—the cranium, thorax, and abdomen. These somatic caves share the same space as the three fields of elixir in qigong and also contain the brain, heart, and enteric brain. They also overlap with distinct branches of the vagus nerve—the frontal vagus connects the head and chest; the lower vagus connects the belly and head. In the form I practice, we place our hands on and center our awareness in the belly, known as the lower elixir field, or Dan Tien. Specifically, this area is the space between the belly button, pelvic floor, and lower back. In Daoist terms, the pelvic bowl is the personal alchemical cauldron where the fire of awareness (yang) is brought to the water of our being (yin). It is easy to understand how the light of our awareness could be analogous to fire but to easily comprehend the symbolic significance of water perhaps takes a little more imagination.

Daoism is sometimes called the way of water, for water exemplifies the flowing nature of the Dao. Water transforms naturally and effortlessly. Daoist's emulate the qualities of water. In the Golden Elixir, the experienced solidity of the body is like ice—full of frozen emotion and fixed beliefs. Fire melts ice, and by keeping the quality of our awareness as bright as fire we melt the experience of the solidity of our body. All bodily and emotional tension is smelted in the cauldron of the pelvic bowl, the part of the body that digests and integrates our experience on many levels. Through persisting in this practice, the actual sensation of heat builds up in the lower belly. If the heat is kept at a constant, this creates a feeling of the body becoming cloudlike. If the heat continues further, this creates an experience of the body transforming into light. The word *light* is both a felt experience of our consciousness as a crystal-clear and boundless luminosity as well as a symbolic icon for emptiness, what Buddhists call Buddha Nature and philosophers call the ground of being.

This process is then reversed, and the light of heaven is returned to the body of Earth. In the form I practice, a major part of this reversal process involves self-massage, which takes the form of pressing specific points on the face, neck, and head; dry washing the face; scrubbing the scalp; and rubbing, massaging, and patting down the trunk and limbs of the body. This brings us back into touch with the physicality of our body and grounds the higher frequencies of luminous consciousness into the lower frequencies of our physical body. The effect is extremely relaxing and enjoyable, giving a sense of radiant contentment. It's also considered an important health measure so that we don't burn up our body essence and float away into the heavenly realms.

When framed within a linear process, the Golden Elixir practice is often described in these steps:

1. Transmuting Jing into qi
2. Transmuting qi into Shen
3. Transmuting Shen into Ming/emptiness
4. Reversing the process

The characters *Jing, qi,* and *Shen* contain a variety of meanings depending on their context. They are coded ways of talking about different states of embodiment. Simply put, Jing is the most material solid aspect of our experience, and Shen is the most imaginative and spiritual aspect of our experience; between the two lies a continuum from embodiment to disembodiment. Qi can be experienced as the interface between body and mind, as well as the capacity for change between body and mind. And so, the Golden Elixir practice follows a natural pattern, which is the transformation between yin and yang.

What we can grasp from this overview of the practice is that it has a strong somatic flavor and explores different modes of consciousness. By resting awareness in the different fields of the body, a deep familiarity of each arising mode of consciousness is established. The solidity of the felt body (known as Jing) is of utmost value, as it is the vessel that carries us toward the light. This contrasts with some forms of meditation, where there is a singular focus on the mind and a disregard for the body. In the Golden Elixir practice, the physicality (Jing) of the body is greatly valued, for it provides the foundation for a stable and calm mind. Being calm is synonymous with being embodied from the lower abdomen, the center of our being.

In the trauma field, there has been much speculation as to the nature of what is called the dorsal vagus, which is the lower branch of the vagus nerve that innervates the abdomen and pelvis. There have been tentative connections between the dorsal vagus nerve and the phenomenon of dissociation, which, as I mentioned before, has received little clinical research. In Golden Elixir practices, and other forms of absorption meditation, there is an intentional type of dissociation from both the body and the self. In both Daoism and Buddhism, a fixed sense of self and identity is considered delusional and a great source of suffering. Too much ego gets in the way of a truthful perception of reality. But it is not only body and self that are transcended, there's also a falling away of all sense of objectivity and subjectivity, time, and space. This might sound paradoxical and, from a clinical viewpoint, dubious or even pathological, but a key feature that differentiates the Golden Elixir from pathological dissociation is a profound sense of safety in the body and equanimity in the mind.

This sense of safety is established in part by lowering the qi, a key and initial aspect of all qigong. The downward flow involves the relaxation of the face, throat, chest, and belly, in this sequence. Like a small pebble sinking to the bottom of a riverbed, our awareness descends through the body and comes to rest at the base of the pelvis. This pathway is the exact parallel of the vagus nerve. In this sense, lowering the qi is a way of self-regulation, of gradually getting in touch with our vagus nerve, and soothing our relationship with our felt body.

This process can be achieved through guiding our internal awareness down into the depths of our body, and it can be more challenging for some than others; therefore, physical touch and massage can greatly assist us. This is where Dien Chan can prove exceptionally helpful in reconnecting our heads with our bodies. When we practice Dien Chan self-massage, we can learn to influence both our vagus nerve and create levels of calmness and comfort in the body that are difficult to achieve through meditation alone. If we tend to be overwhelmed by emotion, whether it be anxiety, depression, or anger, then Dien Chan self-massage can assist us toward integrating these emotions and regaining our individual sovereignty within our heart. By learning how to touch and massage our face and body, we also help bring ourselves back down to Earth, ground ourselves when we feel dissociated, and bring clarity to our senses. This is a good place to begin learning how to perform Dien Chan on ourselves.

FIVE

• •

Touching Faces

Touch can help us feel safe, alive, and real again. It has the potential to turn down the volume on pain, trauma, and anxiety.

STEVE HAINES

Self-massage is something we do naturally, it's the instinctive act of touching our body to relieve discomfort. When we have any kind of itch or discomfort, without any thinking we scratch, press, or rub it. Physical discomfort and tension caused by poor circulation are relieved through touch. This is one of the reasons why bathing and cleansing feels so good—by washing the body and scrubbing ourselves with towels we are secretly giving ourselves a full-body massage.

Mental-emotional discomfort is also relieved through touch, and this is also something we do instinctively—we soothe our troubled minds by touching our body. Often this takes the form of holding our forehead, wringing our hands, or rubbing our thighs. We are usually only half aware of these somatic coping mechanisms, these self-soothing responses to emotional stress. There is a fine line between whether these forms of touch are self-soothing or whether they are just a reflection of internal agitation (like a poker player's "tell"). What tips the balance is the degree to which we can stay present with the sensations in our body. If we can stay present, our touch can convey reassurance like a healing balm, negating the spiraling effects of stress.

The way in which we touch our body is intimately wrapped up in social dynamics. When we cross our arms, we're both projecting a signal outward and self-soothing inward. So much of human communication is nonverbal and relies on body language. When we are with other people and we touch our face, most usually this is a sign that we are in low status—that we're signaling insecurity by hiding our faces. There are, of course, more subtle dynamics to certain gestures, like pensively rubbing one's chin or stroking one's hair, and just like blinking, we instinctively touch our faces an incredible amount of times per day. But it's important to recognize that the simple act of touching one's face is also bound up in all sorts of emotions, self-esteem, and issues of status.

So, the attitude one brings to self-massage is of critical importance. There are two qualities of mind that are very helpful in creating a more powerful change through self-massage. The first is a sense of curiosity, of being open-minded and willing to set aside any prejudgment about what you're doing and just be open to exploration. The second is the sense of love and kindness. We are tending to ourselves in self-massage. The ability to tend to ourselves requires a small amount of tenderness, a recognition that we are deserving of love and kindness. By assuming the slightest of smiles, and letting this hidden smile start to radiate inward, we can generate a flicker of this feeling of love. This is the feeling that we bring into our hands in self-massage.

The hands, knuckles, and fingertips are magnificent tools. To develop skill in massage takes some practice, but fortunately we have a great feedback loop, and so we can learn quickly what feels good for us. Gradually we can tailor our own personalized approach to self-massage by discovering what works best for us. Massage starts in the hands; therefore, we want to bring our energy and attention into our hands to begin. The easiest way to do this it to rub the palms together until there is a little warmth and tingling.

🌸 Self-Care Sequence for Calming the Heart and Soothing the Nervous System

The following sequence brings us in touch with the pathway of the vagus nerve. This technique has the intention of self-soothing, slowing down the nervous system, calming the mind, and bringing clarity to the heart.

1. Place the palms over the eyes. Close the eyes and signal to all the muscles surrounding and behind the eyes to soften and relax.
2. Keep the eyes closed and slowly slide the palms over the temples toward the ears. Press and circle the palms over the ears, then slowly slide the palms downward underneath the jaw and rest the palms over the chest. Listen for the vibration of the heart's pulse through the hands. Gently open the eyes.
3. Let the hands slowly slide downward to the belly. Hold the palms interlocked over the lower belly, just below the belly button. Deepen the breath into the belly and feel the hands expand and contract with the breath.

After performing this sequence, take a little time to notice how you feel. The aim is to create a sense of feeling more comfortable and present within your body. By combining the physical technique with an attitude of kindness and being open to change, we can use this sequence to create a stronger connection to our heart and belly, effectively strengthening our vagal tone. This sequence can be practiced whenever you like and can be repeated a few times or done at half speed.

By stopping and noticing how we feel, we can learn to adapt this technique so that it fits our needs. This could mean skipping the first step and going straight to the ears or even to simply take the holding postures over the heart or belly. Again, although we might assume that Dien Chan concerns solely the face, we are attempting to reconnect our face and head with our heart and belly. This alignment of awareness through the body creates a sense of feeling our whole body together, a vital step to increasing vagal tone. The further one comes to rest in the central axis of the body, the more we can enter a calm space of presence and attunement, a sense of listening with our whole being.

🪷 Self-Care Sequence for Clearing Tension and Refreshing the Mind

The next sequence creates a little more effect, as we go a little deeper into the structures of the body. These techniques are used in a similar fashion to the first sequence, to calm and soothe. They also have the intention of clearing the head of any tension and fuzziness, creating a sense of freshness and clarity. Each step can be performed in five to ten seconds, so the whole sequence can be accomplished in under a minute. Be careful if you are wearing any jewelry. Again, begin by rubbing the palms together to create some warmth.

1. Dry-wash the entire face by rubbing the hands up and down, slowly working outward so the thumbs rub the inside edge of the ears and inward so the pinky fingers rub at the sides of the nose. This can be done anywhere from five to twenty seconds. Press as firmly as feels comfortable, and bring particular attention to feeling any tension release from just underneath the skin.

2. Sweep the palms downward over the face, across the hairline, over the ears, and down the sides of the neck. Sweep a few times each way or as many as feels good.

3. Use scissor hands to rub the inside and outside of the ears five to twenty times.

4. Use the thumb and forefinger to pinch and squeeze from the top of the ears down to the earlobes three times.

5. Use a fingertip to gently cover each earhole, then press down and back and slowly spiral outward three times.

6. Use the knuckles to slowly massage the scalp, from the hairline toward the back of the head.

7. Sweep the fingers through the hair from the front and all the way down the back of the neck, clearing any tension from the head. This can be done with alternating hands or with two hands at the same time.

8. Cross the hands over and squeeze the opposite side of the neck, squeezing and massaging outward to the shoulders and slowly down the arms, finishing with pressing and squeezing the hands together.

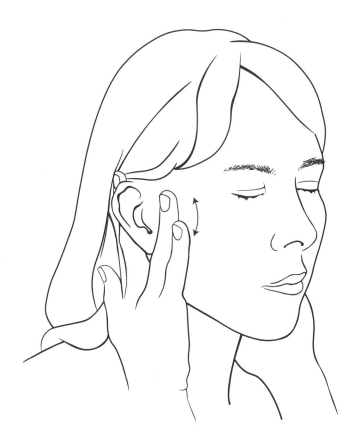

Figure 5.1. Step 3, scissor hands

Again, take time after this massage to notice how you feel. Because these techniques are more active and vigorous, they can boost the circulation through your head, neck, and face, creating a sense of warmth and energy. The intent is both to create a sense of being enlivened and also to clear feelings of physical or energetic stagnation. The sequence can be simplified and adapted, with any one step capable of offering help.

These two basic sequences can be used to remarkable effect. Once you become comfortable with the massage techniques you can adapt them to fit your needs. These simple and quick techniques can help reduce anxiety and stress and increase our sense of feeling at home in the body. They can be used for grounding and stability or to bring clarity and freshness to our perception and can easily be performed at any time of the day and repeated as often as feels good.

The more we can pay attention to how this kind of self-massage affects us, the more we can fine-tune the techniques to create more specific effects on our health. The act of paying attention is perhaps the biggest part of the puzzle, because the ability to feel inside the body can also create change in the body. We can also develop more receptivity to the specific points and areas of the face and deepen our awareness for how they relate to all aspects of our health, emotion, and personality. Dien Chan is a healing system with maps that plot out these relationships. By learning to understand the principles and functions of these points and maps, we can empower our self-healing capacity.

Before we delve in to more nuanced self-massage techniques, let's explore the underlying principle of resonance that enables the healing potential of Dien Chan.

SIX

· ·

Indra's Net of Jewels

Slowly Indra discovered that many worlds were folded away in that empty room, worlds of which he knew nothing.

ROBERTO CALASSO, *KA.*

There is an image from the great Indian world myth of a vast net of jewels that stretches out beyond the farthest reaches of space. It is known as Indra's Net, for he was the god responsible for breaking open the world and unleashing what is called knowledge. Indra was the king of the Devas, the angelic beings, and as such, he adorned each intersection of each thread on this net with a beautiful jewel. Because of the vastness of this net, it contains an infinite number of jewels.

This mythical image is relevant to Dien Chan and Chinese medicine for one subtle detail—if one was to look closely into a single jewel on Indra's net, the shining clarity of the jewel contains within it a reflection of every single other jewel on the net. Each part contains within it a reflection of the whole.

Like a mirror that endlessly reflects itself, Indra's Net is an allusion to the hidden nature of our body and our world. It describes a reality that is entirely connected and interwoven at every level, implying that

81

the way in which everything is connected is not simply mechanistic or linear. This is only the outer appearance of things. Rather, Indra's Net conceives a notion of a reality in which this connectivity is one of co-arising, instantaneous resonance and mutual reflection, an entirely different process that tends to be highly challenging and counterintuitive to linear thinking. It requires a type of fractal thinking that maintains coherence while beholding multiple layers of truth. It takes some real mental gymnastics to truly get your head around! Similar to a sophisticated appreciation of mythical imagery, Indra's Net does not simply represent one idea alone but instead contains all sorts of hidden meanings and implications.

For instance, time, space, and consciousness are thought to have a fractal and holographic nature. Within each moment and point in time and space contains the whole. This leads one into all sorts of philosophical quagmires. But on a more pragmatic level, our human body is also like a net of jewels, with the smallest part of the body connected to, in concert with, and reflecting the greater whole. This is the premise of reflexology—the whole body can be accessed through a single part. Likewise, our personhood as a whole is in resonance with the even greater wholes that we are in turn embedded within. Discovering our sense of wholeness brings us toward a resonance with a universal wholeness.

This understanding of inter-being emerged in many ancient traditions and indigenous cultures. It reflects a wonderfully dynamic approach to living within unfathomably complex systems. Perhaps it stemmed from a deep form of listening to the natural world, for underneath the immediate appearances of things we can learn to perceive a deeper symbiosis within nature, to perceive the trophic cascades that interconnect our ecology. Instead of framing ourselves only as isolated individuals, we can see that on a more fundamental level we exist as a fluid network of contingent relationships. We can feel our life, breath, and heartbeat as an expression of a larger process, connected through our relationships, socially and ecologically.

If we look farther into one of Indra's jewels and we see all the other jewels reflected within it, we can then look closer into the reflection and see that within each reflected jewel is yet another dazzling display of the whole net. And so, by extending our vision we'll bring forth an ever expanding fractal net of reflection.

This vision of fractal entanglement has its conceptual roots in the Vedas, which are some of humanity's oldest texts. It has trickled down through many cultural histories and has seemingly emerged independently around the globe. The image of reality described by Indra's Net was adopted by one of the most renowned historical schools of Buddhism, the Chinese fifth-century Hua Yan, or Flower Adornment, school. Specifically, the Indian Sanskrit Avatamsaka Sutra, from which Hua Yan derives, describes the actual awakening experience of the Buddha as a direct realization of the world as Indra's Net. Rather than describing the specific insights about life and the nature of suffering, which crystallized in the wake of his night under the Bodhi Tree, his pivotal awakening experience, named the Ocean Seal Samadhi, describes all reality as an oceanic mirroring. This image of infinite reflection is later epitomized as Indra's Net.

However, in Chinese culture this vision of all-encompassing inter-penetration predates Buddhism and was known as ganying, a term that not only tells of inter-being at all levels of life but also of a resonance between each mirrored reflection.[1] Ganying translates literally as "stimulus-response." A more encompassing translation could be "universal resonance." It is the underlying principle that shows how the whole body can be reflected on the palm of the hand, sole of the foot, ear, tongue, pulse, abdomen, or, in Dien Chan's case, over the contours of our face.

The concept of ganying was the precursor to the development of yin-yang theory, organ-channel theory, and five element theory, which together constitute the foundational pillars of Chinese medicine. These theories took shape in China between 500 BCE and 200 CE, so ganying is very old indeed. It is the ancient shamanic foundation of acupuncture, reflexology, and all holistic practices derived from Classical Chinese Medicine. Understanding the tangible workings of ganying is central to understanding Dien Chan and Chinese medicine.

Ganying describes how the world changes. The Yi Jing, or Book of Changes, which is the great wellspring of Chinese culture, can be thought of as an exposition of ganying. In the old text known as the *Shih-shuo Hsin-yu,* the renowned monk Hui Yuan is asked, "What is the essence of the Book of Change?" He answers, "ganying is the essence of the Book of Change."[2]

Therefore, the concept of ganying is the key to understanding the correlative cosmology that underpins both Chinese culture and medicine. Gaining insight into this subtle process is relevant for understanding Dien Chan and also for understanding the nature of change and healing in our wider lives.

This old vision of resonance and regeneration, which is wonderfully illustrated by Indra's Net of Jewels, has been paralleled in modern times by the mathematician and polymath Benoit Mandelbrot. His work defined what we now call fractals, self-repeating patterns that occur at every scale in the universe.

Within the world of fractal study, the most often repeated pattern contains a specific geometry known as the Golden Ratio or the Golden Spiral, and we can find it both throughout the proportions of our own face and bodies and throughout nature on every scale. It can be seen in the leaves of plants, roots of trees, courses of rivers, shapes of coastlines, and even in more ephemeral processes in nature, such as the branching of lightning strikes and in forest fires. The Golden Ratio, which is also known by the number phi, can be seen on the microcosmic scale in the spiral structure of our DNA and on the macrocosmic scale within the clustering of galaxies. It is truly breathtaking how this mathematical phenomenon connects all of life.

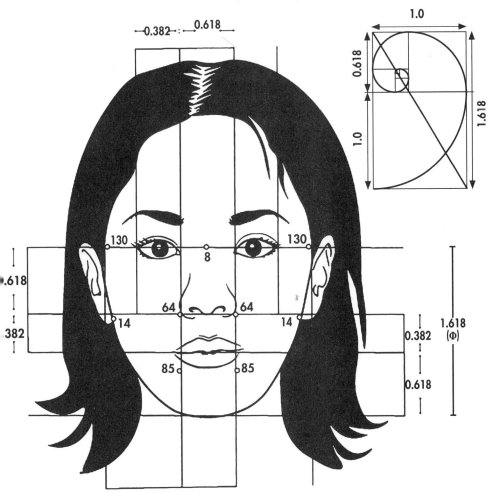

Figure 6.1. The Golden Ratios of the human face and the alignment with Dien Chan points. This face is actually a composite of 100 real-life faces, which in all ethnicities average out to Golden Mean proportions throughout.

The reason these patterns are seen everywhere is that they form the most efficient trajectory for growth and regeneration. This is the hidden code behind our bodies' self-healing power. It also happens to create a unique relationship between each part of a system and its whole.[3] This relationship is expressed in mathematics, and also in the experiential yearning and longing toward wholeness. This relationship has been exploited by Chinese medicine and Dien Chan so that a person can be

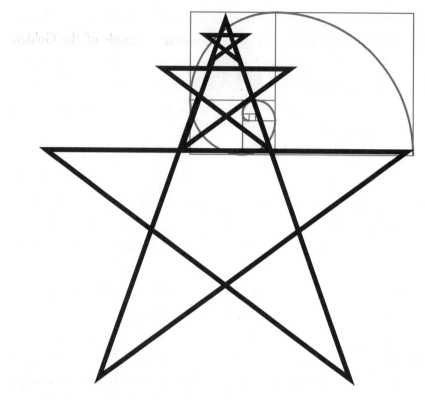

Figure 6.2. The Golden Ratio and
fractal qualities of the pentagram

prompted toward the most optimal path toward wholeness and healing. Many of the most important acupuncture and Dien Chan points align with the Golden Ratio proportions on the body. In this sense, the healing of disease and emotional distress happens by virtue of our bodies' inherent ability to grow, regenerate, and evolve.

If we consider five element theory, which is at the heart of Chinese medicine, we'll clearly see that it's describing a cyclical fivefold pattern between the elements, and for this reason is more accurately called five phase theory. It is descriptive of a symbolic process of change, not of fixed elements. The movement between these phases is organic, fractal, and nonlinear, meaning it cannot be reduced into a simple cause-and-effect mechanism. The geometric symbol of the pentagram illustrates this regenerative cycle clearly. What many don't notice is that each angle and proportion of the pentagram is an exact example of the Golden Ratio, and so five phase theory could be described as a reflection of the fractal nature of life. It is a symbolic map of nature's regenerative code. Each phase is said to be in resonance with emotions and virtues, body tissues, and organs.

Rather than seeing these correspondences as being fixed or essential aspects of each phase, five phase theory points toward an understanding that they only exist in resonance and relation to one another. Like Indra's Jewels, they have a fractal quality, which means that within each element are contained all elements. Each spoke of the pentagram's five sides branches off into another pentagram.

When we consider how five phase theory is applied to healing, there is a particular emphasis on a medicine or treatment not being something that's external to the body but rather as something that is catalyzed inside the body. This is particularly the case with acupuncture, massage, and types of reflexology, like Dien Chan. Resonance, balance, and harmony are emphasized over more forceful techniques like purging, eliminating, or extracting disease because what is being catalyzed by acupuncture and reflexology is nature's intrinsic power for regeneration.

It's important to note that sometimes the body isn't capable of healing all by itself, in which case things like surgical intervention, herbs, antidotes, and medication are entirely necessary. However, it is greatly underestimated how much natural healing power is available to our mind-body, and so for many health issues, as well as for preventive medicine, Dien Chan and other similar healing practices have incredible benefit. They are also much gentler and don't harbor the risks and side effects of over-the-counter medications or cut-and-burn-style medicine.

It's very tempting to see the catalyst toward healing within the metaphor of a machine, as in we press a point that then mechanically triggers a nerve response and a concordant response in blood and hormone circulation. This is the easiest way to understand both acupuncture and

Dien Chan from a reductionist and mechanical viewpoint, as basically tricking the brain through the activation of different types of nerves that release the body's natural painkillers and boost blood circulation to different areas of the body. There is solid research to prove these mechanisms exist.[4]

When our nervous system is first developing in utero, there is a reciprocal innervation among all the mirrored aspects of the body, creating a map in the brain that connects our hands with our feet, our elbows with our knees, our shoulders with our hips, and so on. This map can be manipulated through acupuncture and Dien Chan to release the body's healing chemicals and increase blood circulation to targeted areas of the body.

However, this mechanical explanation is only the outer appearance of healing, it doesn't account for the full potential of acupuncture or Dien Chan, which can dramatically change our sense of embodiment, our emotions, and even the deeper structures of our spiritual lives, such as our self-worth or self-compassion. If we recognize that Dien Chan is prompting our innate capacity and impetus for growth and healing, we can start to see how it can in turn affect all aspects of our life.

To fully grasp Dien Chan, we must realize that nerves and hormones are only part of the picture. The nervous system and hormonal system are vitally important but nevertheless just constitutive parts of this greater process. The regenerative power of nature is at work inside all of us and brings all these different parts of our health together into a cohesive whole. If we reduce health to only one aspect of our body, such as the nervous system or the brain, we miss the bigger picture and risk underestimating our intrinsic power for self-healing.

This begs the question: How do we frame the big picture, the totality of our health? How do we envision every little aspect of our mind-body as a cohesive whole? How do we frame ourselves as a whole person when we are constantly changing and growing into something new?

The reductionist viewpoint might suggest that we are only our bodies and brains, that consciousness is simply an epiphenomenon of our brain, and that mental health is secondary to the primacy of our physical health. This view can be effective when focusing only on the particulars of specific diseases or parts of our body. But it misses the big picture—that we are more than the sum of our parts. We are more than just who we think we are. By this I mean our wholeness co-arises in relationship with the world around us—our family, community, and the living, flowering ecology around us. We are an open whole, evolving, and ever-changing in concert with the world. And given the right environment and circumstances, our bodies will heal entirely by themselves. However, this personal movement toward wholeness, regeneration, and healing is itself part of a greater process within nature. It's not simply that our immediate environment is a factor in our health but rather that the same spark that keeps our hearts beating is at work in the turning of the seasons; we share in the same life.

This shared connection between all parts of our body and the whole, and between our personhood and the greater wholes in which we are embedded; this connection occurs through resonance, ganying. Like Indra's Jewels, it's a mutual co-arising rather than a linear chain reaction. And this resonance underwrites not only all the physical processes of healing but also moves us toward connecting with a primordial wholeness.

This is where things become slightly contentious, because when we start to imagine reality as a whole, this teeters us out into the ineffable and unfathomable. We're broaching into the domain of the sacred—what some consider holy. And because there is so much opinion and spiritual conviction surrounding this topic, talking about nature as a unified whole can bring up some charged feelings. Speaking of such grand things inevitably opens us to the vulnerability of what we do not know, which can be an affront to both atheists and devout religionists alike. It can feel safer to have a certainty of opinion rather than to admit that we don't know what the wholeness of reality might imply.

In traditional Chinese cosmology, the wholeness of reality is sometimes captured by the word Dao, meaning "the Way," and was originally symbolized by the image of a wheel, implying that the Dao is not a fixed path but rather an ever-turning process. Additionally, any mention of the Dao is always given with the caveat: the Dao that can be spoken of is not the true Dao. This is the first line of the Dao De Jing, the foundation of Daoist culture, and gives space for the presence of uncertainty. What we can take from these two ideas is that the wholeness of reality is not a completed thing we exist within but rather is a process that is always changing, unfolding, opening. Closed systems incline toward entropy and degradation; open systems incline toward regeneration. By being open to change, by being open wholes, we can participate and move toward intimacy with the wholeness within nature. This is the way of healing and regeneration that underlies the spiritual vision of Chinese medicine.

Just as modern medicine is long divorced from philosophy and the spiritual imagination, Chinese medicine is married to a spiritual vision of life. In this vision, our physical health is downstream from our mental, emotional, and spiritual health. In turn, our mind and consciousness are also seen as constitutive parts of a greater whole. Going deeper, consciousness itself is considered an intrinsic aspect of nature—human consciousness is embedded within a greater encompassing, nonhuman consciousness.

However, the ancient seers of the Indus Valley and China did more than just conceptualize and philosophize. They directly experienced what is called nondual consciousness, or the *heart of the Dao.* Through meditation they experienced the wholeness of the cosmos as entirely nonpersonal but at the same time with a sense of boundless presence. This blossoming of nondual consciousness in India and China shaped their cultures, philosophy, psychology, and medicine in a profoundly different way from Western cultures. It provided the deep framework for their healing practices and vision of health.

In the classical tradition of Chinese philosophy and medicine, the essential vitality of human health is termed Shen Ming, the illumination of spirit. This is what infuses our body with the impulse toward growth and regeneration. Shen Ming is descriptive of the resonance that takes place between our personhood and nature as a whole. Our personal relationship with nature as a whole shapes how we move through life and how we grow, regenerate, and heal. The greater our attunement with the wholeness in nature, the more optimal our health will be and the greater our capacity for self-healing.

But, practically speaking, how can we relate to the wholeness of nature in a nonabstract way? This is the great task of living well, for as Indra's Net suggests, the whole is available in each and every part. Every relationship we have, within ourselves, our family, ancestors, friends, and strangers—with all that's considered animate and inanimate— reflects an opportunity to align with wholeness and healing.

To begin to behold this can be overwhelming. Usually, we become fatigued when our capacity for relationship is stretched too far. However, regardless of who we are or what we think, humans have a natural reset button that brings us back in resonance with wholeness. This is called sleep, and why sleep is so paramount for healing. Sleep is the state where our mind-body most readily heals, regenerates, and restores our vitality. Deep sleep and dreaming bring us back in touch with Shen Ming. This tunes us back into the song of the world. As the medical doctor and acupuncturist Edward Neal describes:

> Shenming is a special organising illumination around which life processes organise themselves. In classical Chinese the term for the lights of the stellar heavens and the organising illumination of the human body are both called "*shenming*." Because *shenming* is understood to be a prerequisite for the organisation of life, it is also seen to hold the power needed to reform the body along the lines of its original template.[5]

The big questions then arise, which are, besides improving our quality of sleep, how do we access our inherent Shen Ming? What is the real nature of this nondual awareness? And how exactly does it influence our health? The Zen way of phrasing this asks: What is my original face?

In answering these questions, we must recognize that our normal language and thinking has its limitations, for we are grasping at a phenomenon that is both within human experience and at the same time beyond. Terms like Shen Ming, nondual awareness, or mind-at-large are best thought of as simple placeholders. Additionally, our English language carries a strong metaphysical prejudice regarding the nature of mind and matter. It encodes us with intuitive assumptions about the solidity of the world, what Whitehead called "the fallacy of misplaced concreteness."

We tend to think of the physical world as composed of separate things, or as just a bunch of atoms randomly bouncing off one another, whereas both our current science and the old ways of seeing point to a different picture—that of Indra's Net, a vast co-arising web of interdependent relationships. Keeping this in mind, I would suggest we can begin talking about this subject by pointing toward two possible interpretations of the wholeness of nature or mind-at-large.

The first is commonly described in Buddhism as emptiness. Like a unitive background to all of reality, emptiness is sometimes described experientially as *clear light* or as the *bliss void*. One of the key insights of the Buddha was that both our personal mind and consciousness as a universal phenomenon are, at a fundamental level, empty. Empty of an intrinsic self—just wide open, spacious, and clear. The great twelfth-century Chinese Zen master Hong Zhi gave us this description:

> We all have the clear, wondrously bright field from the beginning . . .
> its brightness doesn't shine out but can be called empty and inherently radiant. Its brightness, inherently purifying, transcends causal conditions beyond subject and object. Subtle but preserved, illu-

mined and vast, also it cannot be spoken of as being or nonbeing, or discussed with images or calculations.[6]

It is important to recognize that emptiness is different from nothingness, as this has great bearing on our relationship with nihilism and how we discover meaning in our lives. If we believe everything is nothing, and that life is all for nothing, this does not infuse our life with much vitality, enthusiasm, or good-heartedness. This isn't what's being referred to when Buddhists describe the nature of the mind and the world as empty. Rather, emptiness describes what might be called the flavor of liberation, for it frees us from despair and nihilism. When our mind touches this ground level of emptiness, the notion of our mind disappears, there is no constraint of individual identity. This gives a sense of being momentarily free from the afflictions and pain of life. From an individual perspective, this sense of personal oblivion might seem scary, but the people who taste emptiness don't report fear but instead a deep and profound sense of relief and refuge.

Now, it might be assumed that only meditation experts can experience emptiness, as though it's a VIP zone for spiritual masters. And although people who engage in self-inquiry, meditation, or contemplative practices can sometimes become more familiar with the experience of emptiness, by its definition, emptiness is something in which we are already embedded and suffused. We are never really disconnected from this primordial field of consciousness. It is what we return to every night in deep sleep. But, we can get confused and embroiled in ways of thinking that assert a certain forcefulness of identity, and this can dampen the connection to this empty field. Experiencing and becoming embroiled in strong emotions, desires, and aversions this can often create a fixed mind-set—a sense of solidity of the ego self—which can dampen the full expression of Shen Ming. Therefore, the quality of our conscious and emotional life plays a key role in all aspects of our health and our capacity for self-healing.

This is an important takeaway from this interpretation of emptiness—our health is downstream of our emotional lives.

The second interpretation of mind-at-large describes all phenomena as emerging from an infinite web of conditions. This is sometimes called the tenet of interdependent origination—that nothing exists in pure isolation. Rather than frame emptiness as some separate realm of enlightenment, this interpretation describes the entirety of the world, including our bodies and minds, as existing only through contingent relationships.

Life is a co-arising field of reflection and resonance, the vision that underpins both Indra's Net of Jewels and ganying, universal resonance. It suggests that even though mind, body, and world are impermanent and ever-changing, there is still a principle and pattern in the deep background of reality, and this shapes the growth, development, and regeneration of life.

This principle of interdependence points to all of life as being holographic. Holograms, like the ones we see on credit cards, have an often unknown feature—when they are cut in half, each half contains the whole image. When they are quartered, each quarter contains the whole image. This happens regardless of how many times the image is split, although the resolution becomes weaker the smaller you go. This same feature is described by Indra's Net—every little part of life, on every level, interpenetrates and contains the whole.

The Avatamsaka Sutra describes this fractal vision in endlessly weaving poetic verses, such as:

> In a single atom there are untold lotus worlds.
> In each lotus world are untold Chief of Goodness
>   Buddhas.
> Pervading the entire cosmos and every atom therein.
> Worlds, becoming, subsisting, and decaying, are
>   measureless, unspeakable in number.

The point of a single atom is boundless, containing
measureless lands therein.[7]

One of the implications of this interpretation of emptiness is that all of life can be seen as adornment, as a display of beauty. This bears relevance for how we conduct our emotional lives and how we discover meaning in our lives. Instead of concluding that the solution to life's suffering is to diminish all emotion and escape the world of bodily forms, we are presented with a more romantic option—affirming the love, bliss, and beauty of life.

Whereas some people might dismiss the vision of Indra's Net as taking the interconnectivity of life to the level of the absurd, resulting in meaninglessness, this misses a vital point. Our relationship to the whole can flourish when we savor life, when we relish and make space for beauty and wonderment. Creating an orientation toward beauty in how we relate to other people and the world around us can attune us to the wholeness in ourselves and the world. Not only does this affect the meaningfulness and zest we have for life but also our ability to heal, regenerate, and grow as people.

I believe one of the reasons Hua Yan Buddhism is held in such high esteem is that is strikes this middle balance between asceticism and adornment, which has such relevance for meaning making and spirituality in the messy festival of urban societies. It also points to an important clue in how emotions relate to our health, in that there is a great power in certain emotions for aligning ourselves to Shen Ming and self-healing. We'll explore these implications further in the coming chapters.

Benoit Mandelbrot may have sparked the modern exploration of the holographic universe, but there have been many other highly esteemed scientists and thinkers who have seriously entertained this vision of life. A special mention must be given to the genius of David Bohm and

Wolfgang Goethe, who drew inspiration from an intuitive vision of the wholeness of nature.

In more recent times the eminent theoretical physicist Carlo Rovelli has spearheaded a view of life that is fundamentally interdependent and relational. He says, "The properties of any entity are nothing other than the way in which that entity influences others. It exists only through its interactions. Quantum theory is the theory of how things influence each other. And this is the best description of nature that we have."[8]

The microbiologist Kriti Sharma has written with striking clarity how it is not just in the abstracted realm of quantum mechanics that interdependence defines the world. It's also a key feature of our human biology. Her work details how signal transduction—that is, the cellular process within our bodies that enables our perception and experience of life—is not only a process of interaction but also of interdependence. She writes:

> We are not radically separate from what we commonly conceive as "external reality." We are always in touch with reality and are completely at home in the world. The world is not a place that is created once and then waits for us to discover it. The world comes into being moment by moment, dependent upon our participation. This is why our being in the world—our participation in its making—is so central to its continued creation, and this is part of the goodness of living.[9]

Sharma describes how our senses are in active participation with the world and how this relationship dispels any notion that we are ever in true isolation. Instead, our sensual contact with everything we see and touch is calling forth the world around us. This is a marvel that imbues life with a sense of belonging, that we are not only part of this world around us, but integral to its creative and continuous renewal. However, the interdependence of our sense perception with the world around us is not only happening outside of us, it's also infused within us, within our bodies. In its essence, Dien Chan plays on this resonant interior web, what one might call our personal Net of Indra. By learning the self-healing practices of Dien Chan we can discover these holographic dynamics within our face and being. We can start to unveil our holographic self.

The fractal growth in nature displays a movement toward wholeness. Greater and greater wholes. We are part of this movement and impulse toward wholeness. This impulse drives our growth, regeneration, and self-healing. Dien Chan taps in to and realigns us with this impulse. The beauty of Dien Chan is that it maps out the areas where our life vitality becomes stuck, and through the use of massage provides a way of releasing these stuck patterns. Many of these points and areas on the face align with emotional expressions and with the golden proportions of the face. By stimulating and releasing these points, we open a window of opportunity to change our expression of life and open toward growth, wholeness, and healing.

The maps of Dien Chan show that the face is like a jewel on Indra's Net. Within the face the whole body is reflected in myriad ways. These different reflections connect part and whole and can be used to prompt different aspects of our health toward healing. In the next chapter we'll explore these maps and points so that we can begin forming pragmatic skills in Dien Chan.

When we develop a self-care practice in Dien Chan, this brings a feeling of self-soothing and coming home to the body—of feeling grounded and settled—both emotionally and physically. By becoming sensitive to the holographic dimension of our mind-body—what might be called the holographic self—we can also learn to regulate specific aspects of our physiology and open ourselves toward self-healing and wholeness.

SEVEN

· ·

Maps of Healing

I am large. I contain multitudes.

WALT WHITMAN

The face is a holo-map for every aspect of our mind-body. Each part of the face contains hidden pathways that can connect to and influence all aspects of our body and mind. In Vietnam, Professor Bui Quoc Chao discovered more than twenty-five different maps, each showing the correlations between the face and various aspects of our body. By stimulating the active areas of the face, we can then affect change in the correlating parts of our body or mind. We know when an area or point is active because it feels especially sensitive. This active area is sometimes called the living point, or in acupuncture the *ah-shi* point (ouchy point). The heightened sensitivity of these points has been discovered to create a stronger balancing and healing response in the body.

The face is one of the most sensitive parts of the body; it is responsive to incredibly small amounts of pressure, and we can clearly differentiate touch on the face from one *millimeter* to the next. Dien Chan relies on this sensitivity to track where there is stagnation in the body or mind. A point the size of a sesame seed can feel normal, whereas the slightest shift in position can elicit a much stronger response, either through physical tenderness or emotional reaction.

Professor Bui researched how these living points would elicit healing effects in his patients, and over the years he mapped out more than three hundred points on the face that are associated with specific effects on our health and physiology. Some of these points are used to affect the various organs, address pain in different parts of the body, and influence whole-body processes such as sleep, digestion, temperature, and anxiety. By becoming familiar with the maps and points of the face, we can learn to balance and improve all aspects of our health. As a self-care practice, Dien Chan can also help us to get to know and come to appreciate our holographic self, which can act as both a preventive health measure, creating improved emotional regulation, and a proactive psychosocial measure toward a more present and felt sense of wholeness and inter-being with the people and life around us.

It's important to realize that these maps show potential connections that may differ from person to person. Each face is different and holds tension and emotion in nuanced ways, which alter the application of these holo-maps. We all share our expressions to a certain degree; therefore, there are protocols and go-to points for certain ailments contained within Dien Chan practice. However, the more complex the imbalance, the more tailored our approach should become. This doesn't mean that the more complex our health problems are, the more complex our treatment should be. On the contrary, it's often by taking a simpler yet more focused approach that we can create a stronger healing response.

We tailor our approach in part by becoming familiar with the Dien Chan maps and learning the points and areas of correspondence that are relevant to our needs. We also need to step beyond the anatomical body and connect to the felt body, which means becoming present to the particular feelings and nuances that can be discovered through self-massage. This requires listening into our body and being curious so as to discover the points and areas that are most active and sensitive on our face. Physical sensitivity is the easiest to feel, but emotionally active points are just as common on the face. Often, they are intertwined. Sometimes they are hidden behind masks, and it's only through close attention to our body that we can unveil them. This takes a willingness to slowly and patiently feel into our body with curiosity, honesty, and a degree of courage.

❧ Exploring the Face

We instinctively touch our face to soothe emotion. Are we able to shift from doing this unconsciously to touching with care and intent? Tentatively explore your face from jawline to hairline, ears to nose, and notice if touching any point or area on the face elicits a feeling or emotion. Regardless, if a point or area feels physically or emotionally sensitive, the best way to release these points is to have a sense of giving in to them, of internally relaxing in response to the pressure. This is best done by remaining calm, present, and not bracing against the pressure. If there is any subtle bracing, then bring this into your awareness and see if you can relax the face. The pathway of release is downward, so using the out breath to soften and relax downward is a helpful tool to consciously support Dien Chan. This is actually something we instinctively do in massage—we take a long sigh to help release from the inside.

PRIMARY MAPS OF DIEN CHAN

The primary map that lays the foundation for the art of Dien Chan can be seen in figure 7.1.

This map overlays representations of two bodies over the center of the face. This is the easiest map to use to begin seeing the connections between parts of the face and aspects of the body. An easy way to intuitively understand this map is to look at the area above the eyebrows. As you can see, this corresponds with the shoulders and upper arms. These two parts of the body are where most people consistently hold stress and

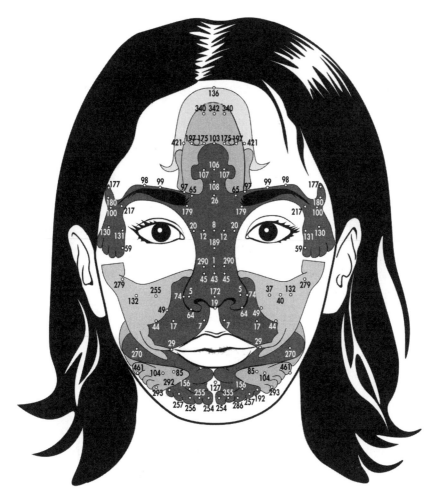

Figure 7.1. The full body map

tension—in the shoulders and on the brow of the face. So, by squeezing and releasing tension from the brow, this in turn will release the shoulders. The more specific points and areas of tenderness on and above the eyebrows can help clear many types of neck and shoulder pain. If there is any pain, injury, illness, or imbalance in the body, we can stimulate the corresponding parts on the face and induce a healing effect.

The other key map in Dien Chan is seen in figure 7.2 on page 102, which displays the major organs of the body over the face. There are

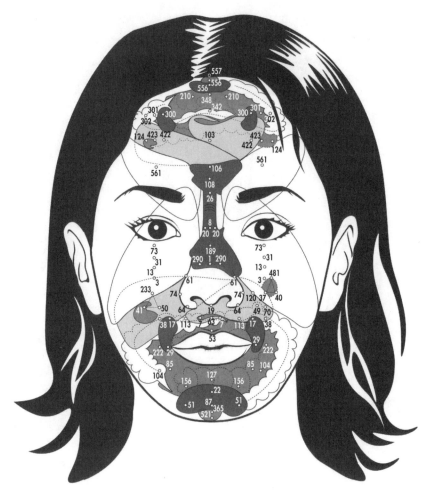

Figure 7.2. The organ map

two reflections, with one underneath the level of the brow and a second inverted and overlaid onto the forehead. So, with this map there are always two options when looking to work with an organ. If, for instance, one wants to affect the liver, the options could be to massage the area below the right cheek or to massage the area in the center of the forehead above the right eyebrow. Either the whole area can be massaged or small specific points in the area can be stimulated. This doubling up of the images introduces us to the dynamic options that are made available through Dien Chan. Because there are so many maps, there are multiple ways of finding the active and effective points on the face.

DIRECT AND INDIRECT POINTS
FOR CONNECTING TO THE VAGUS NERVE

If we consider the fundamental importance of the vagus nerve in healing, it's natural to wonder how to activate it through Dien Chan. In the broadest sense, any massage that relaxes the face is touching into the vagus nerve, and so the initial techniques given in chapter 6 have already given us an impression for how to affect our vagal tone. However, there are different entry points for switching into our healing mode. In Dien Chan, we have the options of going to the area on the face where the vagus is most directly accessibleas well as using the holographic map that relates to each cranial nerve. Exploring these two options is a good way to explore the difference between the linear and nonlinear approaches in Dien Chan. One is more direct and mechanical; the other is more oblique and happens through resonance.

❀ Direct Vagus Nerve Stimulation

The most direct point for the vagus nerve is highlighted by the therapy known as vagus nerve stimulation, which attaches an electric current to the point on the surface of the body where the vagus is most accessible. As it happens, this is also where one of the master points of Dien Chan resides, known as point 0 (see figure 7.3 on page 104). The location is just in front of the lower ear, where your finger comes to rest if you open your jaw wide and feel for the space created, just near what is called the tragus. Try to gently stimulate this point and take notice of how you feel. This point is always used at the end of a treatment, for it is said to seal the effect of the treatment into the body. It carries the effect of the treatment down through the body. It can also be used in a singular way to activate the vagus nerve.

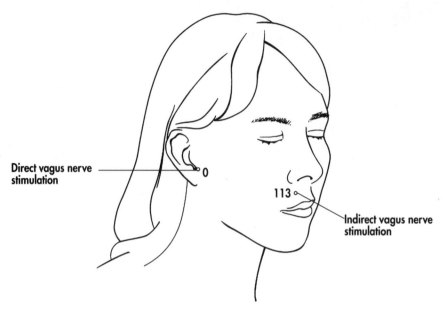

Direct vagus nerve stimulation

0

113

Indirect vagus nerve stimulation

Figure 7.3. Dien Chan points for stimulating
the vagus nerve

❦ Indirect Vagus Nerve Stimulation

The indirect point used to activate the vagus nerve is found by looking at the Dien Chan map that overlays the brain and cranial nerves over the face. Point 113 (see figure 7.3), which is located midway between the outer edge of the nose and the lip, specifically resonates with the vagus nerve. Try stimulating this point by using the middle fingers to press upon both points, gently making small circles. Notice how you feel.

We can use these two points in a broad and quick way to create a change in our nervous system, away from the fight-or-flight response. Learning how to feel the difference between the two points teaches us how to explore the different structural and resonant aspects of our person.

DIEN CHAN SEQUENCES FOR WHOLE-BODY BALANCE AND PREVENTIVE HEALTH CARE

The following two sequences have been created as daily routines for preventive health care. They effectively stimulate all the key areas of the face, which in turn gently signals to all the systems of the mind-body to balance and come to homeostasis. For this reason, they are fantastic for supporting general health and well-being, and can also be used as a simple way to enhance the body's natural healing power.

❈ Bui Quoc Chau's Eight-Step Protocol for Self-Healing and Immune Support

The first sequence was created by Professor Bui specifically to harmonize the organs of the body and to boost lymphatic circulation, thereby supporting the immune system. With each step it is ideal to make thirty-six repetitions. However, one can also perform this sequence quickly with five to ten repetitions and still create a good effect. See figure 7.4 on page 106 for points.

1. Use the tips of the index fingers to rub the line between the inside tip of the eyebrows to the inside corners of the eyes.
2. Use the pad of the middle finger to rub up and down the bridge of the nose and center of the forehead.
3. Use the tips of the index and/or middle fingers to rub along the nasal curve.
4. Use the tips of the index and/or middle fingers to rub along the smile line (the curving line between the nostrils and outer lips).
5. Make a loose fist and use the curve of the index finger to rub the chin.
6. Use the pads of the index fingers to circle around the ears.
7. Use the pads of the index fingers to sweep along the upper lip line.
8. Use the pads of the index fingers to sweep along the middle forehead line.

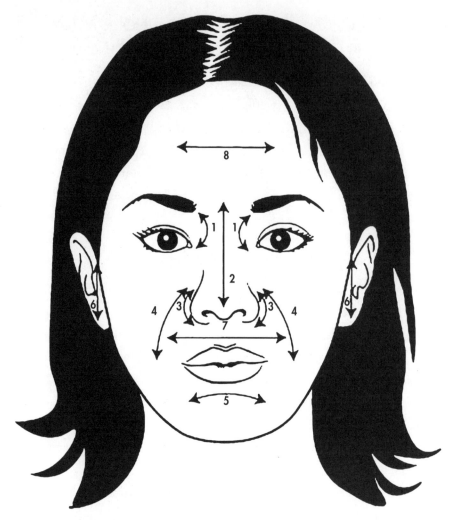

Figure 7.4 Professor Bui Quoc Chau's eight-step protocol

❧ Self-Care Sequence for Emotional and Nervous System Balance

The second sequence offers a way to release both physical and mental tension and to create a sense of balance between the two sides of the brain and body. The first two steps on the eyebrows and ears should be performed for ten to twenty seconds, while the last two steps can be done slightly quicker. See figure 7.5 on page 108 for hand motions.

1. Cross the hands over and use the thumb and forefingers to pinch, press, and squeeze the opposite eyebrows. Work with as much pressure as feels comfortable, from the inside of the eyebrow outward and back.

2. Keep the hands crossed and extend them farther to the opposite ears. Again, pinch, press, and squeeze from the top of the ears to the earlobes, pulling down the earlobes.

3. Use the pinky fingers to press points 26 and 126; both points are on the centerline, with 26 directly above the lips in the center of the philtrum and 126 directly below on the crease line of the chin. As you press the points, use the tip of the tongue to press where the top finger is (just above the teeth) and then where the bottom finger is (toward the chin line). Switch hands and repeat.

4. Bring the palms together in front of the sternum, either clasped or in prayer position. Feel the palms press together, and let your awareness listen to the beating of the heart.

It's helpful to pause and take a snapshot of how you feel before and after each one of these routines. After the massage, the face will feel a bit more alive and sensitive, but pay particular attention to any changes you might feel in your body. The intention for both sequences is to create a change in how you feel—bringing a sense of balance and harmony to our body and mind.

The four different sequences we have explored so far give an easy impression of the effects that Dien Chan self-massage can create. Although the sequences are fairly simple and minimal, this gives us an idea of the potential they have for affecting change in our mind and physiology. Each sequence has a slightly different effect, and they can be adapted and used in whichever way feels best to you. They can be used as much as needed or incorporated into other self-care routines, including washing and bathing, yoga, meditation, breathing practices, and so on.

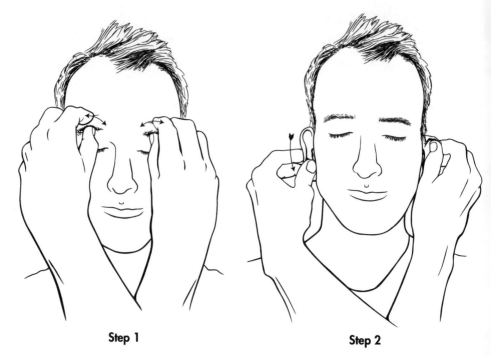

Step 1

Step 2

Figure 7.5. Self-Care Sequence
for Emotional and Nervous
System Balance
Step 1, cross-hands massage
for the eyebrows.
Step 2, cross-hands massage
for the ears.
Step 3, balancing Dien Chan
points 26 and 126.

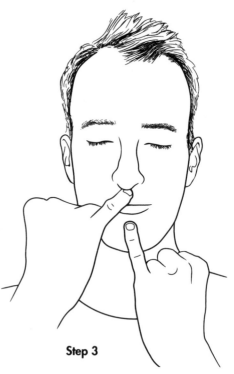

Step 3

❖ ❖ ❖

Dien Chan is an easy and instinctive way of self-soothing and bringing balance to our mind and body. By simply using our hands as our tools we can achieve some remarkable effects, turning around our state of mind and even imbalances in our health. However, the more powerful healing effects of Dien Chan seen in the clinics of Vietnam are achieved via the use of massage tools. The face is exquisitely sensitive, much more so than the back, chest, or legs. The density of nerves that surrounds our mouth, for instance, creates a sensitivity that is attuned to the micromillimeter. For this reason, the width of each fingertip is simply too big to tap in to the nuance that is available in our face.

Initially, back in the late 1970s, Professor Bui used acupuncture needles on the face. The types of needles available at that time were very different from the ultrathin needles used in cosmetic acupuncture nowadays. Subsequently, he realized the treatments did not need to be as painful as acupuncture to elicit a healing response.

By using a massage tool like a thin chopstick or even a toothpick, one could create just as significant a response without the overwhelming sensations that acupuncture can sometimes create. From this discovery he started inventing a whole range of massage tools for different uses and effects in Dien Chan. Generally speaking, the point stimulator is the first and most important tool. Its use is halfway between acupressure and acupuncture. The dozens of other tools can be broadly categorized into either yin (soothing, cooling) or yang (stimulating, warming) effects. There are tools that are specifically designed to rub, tap, cool, comb, and squeeze parts of the face and body, and although people often raise their eyebrows when they see them, each tool can create a certain feeling of pleasure and comfort in the body. (For an exploration into massage tools, see appendix A.) As a healing system, Dien Chan has several principles and set formulas to treat a very wide range of illnesses and disorders. There are also several schools of thought pertaining to different styles of facial reflexology, and there is even a style that is purely cosmetic in function. However, in my experience, one of the most profound effects of Dien Chan is on the mind. This is in part why I've found myself moving toward specializing in stress and trauma. I believe that because Dien Chan emerged from out of the wreckage of war, it is particularly apt in treating the whole spectrum of problems that arise from extreme stress and trauma. It's also my belief that our culture is stumbling blindly through the midst of a great mental health crisis, unrealized and unacknowledged for the most part.

Never before in recorded history have we had such levels of depression, anxiety, and suicide. The crisis is largely the result of stress and trauma, from within people's personal lives and from intergenerational cycles of unresolved trauma. Another important factor is the physiological stress incurred from the pollution that saturates our water, food, soil, and air.

The strain and stress on our ecological and societal environment is deeply connected to this hidden epidemic of stress and trauma. The more we investigate the nature of poor health, pain, and disease, the more interconnections we discover among different systems of the body, mind, lifestyle, and the wider environment. It is often the case that someone's stomach cramps, migraines, or back pain are connected in some way to emotional stagnation, which traces further back to the relational dynamics of our family, social circle, and circumstances.

We have briefly looked into the history of stress and trauma and its entanglement with the nature of consciousness and emotion. Although emotions seem so familiar, being quite literally in our faces, we assume that our science has a clear understanding of their workings. Western culture's theories of consciousness and emotion haven't changed significantly in more than one hundred years—since the time of Darwin. From the traditional Eastern viewpoint, there is also a wide range of opinion about the nature of emotions. Therefore, to avoid stumbling on blindly, we need a reassessment of the nature of emotion and the relationship between our emotions and our health.

EIGHT

. . . .

Emotional History

I live in the facial expressions of the other, as I feel him living in mine.

MAURICE MERLEAU-PONTY

Emotions are not reactions to the world; they are your constructions of the world.

LISA FELDMAN BARRETT

The face has eighty-four little muscles, which differs from the rest of our body's muscles in many ways. The purpose of the muscles in our arms, legs, or back is to enable movement and to support our balance. The body's muscles are innervated via the spine, whereas the face is innervated via the cranial nerves of the head (including the vagus nerve, also known as cranial nerve X).

From an evolutionary standpoint, the original purpose of our face is to enable eating, breathing, and the mediation of our senses. But our face is also inextricably bound up in emotional expression. The facial muscles enable us to communicate our feelings to others, give structure to our language, and are the visual component to our speech. These muscles not only communicate outward, but they also mimic other people's facial expressions, and this subtle mirroring communicates inward, into our internal world. In other words, our muscles allow us to register and internalize the feelings of others, playing a crucial part in empathy. This allows us to orient and harmonize ourselves with other people.

These functions of the face—for emotional communication, language, perception, mimicry, eating, and breathing—all share an underlying feature, the fact that the face bridges between our internal state and our external world. The flow between these two spheres bridges in both directions: our internal state and external world inform each other. For example, consider how the act of squinting our eyes both changes our vision and also communicates emotion to others. From a different angle, consider how our emotional state changes our perception, both of other people and of what is salient in our world around us.

Our face has a unique ability to interface between our sense of self and the world—between emotion and perception.

However, exactly what are emotions? This question might seem simple because we are so familiar with how emotions feel. Anger and joy, sadness and fear—these feelings are like the air we breathe; they suffuse our social environment, giving color to our lives. But to answer this question beyond our personal intuition is no easy task, as much uncertainty remains when it comes to the science of emotion.

Our personal intuition might describe emotion as movement of energy or the brain's reactions to the world. Both the layperson and scientist often start off with similar baseline assumptions when it comes to understanding emotion, but this does not cut the mustard, for if emotion really does play such an important part in our health, we must try our best to expand our frame of vision so that we can begin to account for the current uncertainties.

To really know how emotions arise and fade, and to deeply comprehend the intricacies of their nature, we must step beyond conventional understanding. Only in this way can we start to address the full complexity of the various crises that result from stress and trauma. The typical conventional understanding of emotion is largely based on assumption and has no definitive answers. In fact, the scientific study of emotion is quite contentious, because it often draws one into the mysteries of consciousness and the various cultural foibles surrounding the mind-body relationship.

Emotions are qualitative experiences of one's consciousness. Like other aspects of consciousness, they also have a wide range of physical correlates in our expression and biology. But just like color or taste, we have no explanation for why emotions feel the way they do. There is no scientific explanation that fully describes the suchness of experience. We can say that the taste of an apple or the color of a flower have certain molecular compositions, or that emotions have specific neurological and hormonal centers and pathways, and that these things make our brains ping in a particular way, but this fails to explain the full experiential flavor and complexity of sadness or love. It fails to explain why emotions feel the way they do.

Historically, it has been very challenging to study emotions precisely for this reason—how do we begin to study, measure, and quantify something that is so subjective and qualitative in experience?

In the past, scientists have grappled with this challenge in various ways, but a general consensus developed, which informs our society's typical understanding of emotion. This consensus suggests that emotions result from the brain, or the brain in concert with the endocrine and nervous system. I wouldn't suggest that this assumption is wrong but instead that it presents an oversimplified picture of a process that is more complex than we might suspect. Simplifying such fundamental aspects of our human experience can lead and has led to many warped extrapolations.

For instance, much of the miscommunication, sexism, racism, and dehumanization of the past hundred years is intimately related to such extrapolations about our biology and emotion. The stereotypes of women being innately more emotional, and therefore handicapped from responsible decision making, or that different cultures are innately more or less virtuous—these examples connect back to different periods of scientific theorizing regarding emotion.

Whereas it might be tempting to think we've outgrown such misconceptions, our culture as a whole is still very much confounded by its assumptions and confusion regarding emotions. It can be ever so easy to relegate the issue to the back burner, for it can be overwhelmingly complex trying to comprehend emotion from personal, societal, and cultural standpoints. However, as we are just beginning to recognize the implications for our collective health, there are exciting signs of a change in how our culture-at-large approaches emotion.

This might come as a surprise to you, but the scientific study of emotion has reached a watershed moment. The data we have points toward a new paradigm—a new understanding that has profound significance.[1] Coincidently, this new way of understanding emotion has striking parallels with some of the old wisdom traditions from which Dien Chan and the Golden Elixir stem. Before we explore these parallels, it's worth backtracking over the history of the study of emotion so we can more fully reassess the status quo.

Charles Darwin is the grandfather of the science of physiology and psychology. His theory of evolution redefined what it is to be human and placed us into a familial relationship with animals and our animal nature. He was also the first person to formulate a scientific understanding of emotion, which he established in his book *The Expression of Emotion in Man and Animals* (1872). From the start he drew a parallel between facial expressions and specific emotions. He thought that emotions had to have their source as an evolutionary survival mechanism. With this line of thinking, primitive emotions like fear and rage were the first to develop in our ancient ancestors.

Given that violence has significantly shaped our history and evo-lution, it would make sense that violent emotions could be explained as an evolutionary instinct. However, the question of how our pro-social emotions evolved is not as easy to understand. The evolu-tionary drive to procreate could be thought of as the cause of lust, and the human emotion of love could be seen as simply a by-product of lust. But altruism, compassion, empathy, wonder, and awe—these do not easily square with the survival of the fittest hypothesis. These pro-social emotions proved to be a real problem for Darwin, a prob-lem that was never fully resolved and that had a profound influence on the course of the twentieth century.*

The view that the pro-social emotions were the weak emotions and that the dominance of predatory behavior was entirely natural and necessary—both in the marketplace and in governance—still has clear relevance for our personal and business relationships today. It's the classic dichotomy between getting ahead and getting along, which has shaped the ideological, socioeconomic, and geopolitical battlegrounds throughout the twentieth century.

I would suggest that it's actually a false dichotomy—in the same way we frame our nervous system as existing either in the fight mode or the rest mode, this is an oversimplification of what's going on. The modern explanations tend toward explaining altruism as a covert selfishness, in that we are only kind toward others when there is a personal incentive. They nevertheless frame humans purely as an alpha predator.

---

*The precedent set by Darwin influenced societal governance, politics, marketing, and business. Throughout the twentieth century, we based our social lives on the assumption that the pro-social emotions were a thin veneer shielding our true nature, which is that of the primal emotions of survival—anger, lust, and selfishness. This history is most clearly laid out in the documentary "The Century of the Self" by Adam Curtis (2002), BBC. For a clear investigation of the original issues, see Robert J. Ludwig and Martha G. Welch, "Darwin's Other Dilemmas and the Theoretical Roots of Emotional Connection."

If we instead consider how vital collaboration is for our species, and perhaps use a polyvagal lens of our nervous system, empathy and altruistic behavior can be explained as our default mode. Instead of defining ourselves as essentially selfish predators, there is good evidence that collaboration is the overarching principle that governs human survival. As humans, this is the key to long-term success: to engage in life with a playful openness and kindness rather than seeing life as a fight to the death.

This is what the modern big thinkers such as Steven Pinker, Matt Ridley, David Sloan Wilson, and Rutger Bregman all promote—that we have good reason to believe in the potential for human kindness, collaboration, and optimism over and above human cynicism, selfishness, and cruelty. Unfortunately, however, it is the oversimplified dichotomy of our fight and rest modes that still primarily shapes how we culturally and individually understand our emotions and see ourselves.[2]

Darwin developed his theory of evolution in a very buttoned-up Victorian society. Being rational, having a stiff upper lip, and being in control over one's emotions was already a social virtue, but his theory bolstered the idea that giving in to emotion was a moral weakness akin to becoming a savage animal. It was also seen as an inherently female weakness. The mental illness of hysteria, which reflects the symptoms of what we now call PTSD, was initially diagnosed only in women.

Hyster is Latin for "womb," implying that having a womb is the source of this type of emotional instability, and therefore incapable for men. To be emotional was unmanly and a disgrace to our God-given gift of reason. It's for this reason that the very same symptoms had to be renamed as war hysteria—for the soldiers who survived the trenches of World War I. At the time, these soldiers were seen as weak and lacking a stiff upper lip.

Sigmund Freud was the grandfather of psychology and was greatly influenced by Darwin. His idea of the unconscious and how we repress the socially unacceptable emotions of lust and anger into the unconscious is still widely accepted. In fact, the original ideas that Darwin had about emotion have remained nearly unchanged in 160 years, which is truly remarkable.[3] Either he was spot on, or we have collectively ascribed to an epic level of cognitive dissonance and bias.

Consider how much has changed in the fields of biology and physics, whereas our understanding of emotion and consciousness appears to be culturally locked into a Victorian assumption that we must master our emotions with divine reason—like enslaving an animal. The idea that emotional skills and mental health can be formally taught in school would sound alien and unnecessary for many people. This is particularly relevant when it comes to our emotional development as children and the way in which we learn the social language of emotions from our parents. Many people would assume that kids just naturally learn these skills, and it's true that they are incredibly impressionable. But what happens when they also inherit our collective trauma?

Are babies born with genetically encoded emotional instincts like fear and anger? Or do we gradually learn emotions from our parents or caregivers? These two questions reflect two different assumptions—the first is that emotions arise from a physiological mechanism, as if there is a gene that governs the expression of fear. The second is that emotions are stable things we all share and experience in the same fashion.

These assumptions are taken as pre-givens for modern people, but there is significant evidence that other cultures and indigenous peoples engage with emotion in entirely different ways. Not only are there entirely different concepts and words for emotions in different cultures, like the German *schadenfreude* or the Brazilian *saudade,* but the way in which emotions are embodied and how they inform people's behavior also differ from one culture to the next. This is the inconvenient truth that Darwin, Freud, and the mainstream view they created, has been embattled with.

Since the times of Darwin, we haven't found a testable hypothesis that can prove emotional instincts in newborns. It's not simply that we can't find a universal expression of anger or fear in babies, but we still have no definite scientific understanding of how and why empathy and love arise. However, within the first one to two years it's clear that infants can express empathy, seeking to calm and relieve suffering in others.[4] Interestingly, within the first twenty-four hours babies have been shown to mimic the faces that are looking at them—to play copycat of the facial expressions we project. Although it seems abundantly clear that a baby is in need when it's crying, can we be so certain that babies experience the same emotions of fear, anger, and joy that we are so familiar with?

This hints toward two aspects of the study of emotion that require attention. The first is that emotions are subjective; they are qualitative and therefore can't be accurately measured or quantified. This has meant that any talk of emotion has historically lacked scientific validity, which in turn reinforced the status quo of seeing emotions as a sign of weakness—of being vague and lacking control.

The second is the more modern tendency to categorize emotions in broad brushstrokes—what is called emotional essentialism. This tendency assumes there is an inherent essence to each of the basic emotions. This lack of nuance doesn't account for how we can experience a massive range of feelings within the word *anger,* such as irritation, agitation, disgruntlement, sulking, fury, enmity, feeling tetchy, or the burning desire for vengeance.

While we might conform to our cultural description of being angry, inside we might also be awash with anger, fear, and grief—alongside hints of nostalgia, envy, and anxiety. It would be so simple if a single emotion had a single corresponding pathway in the brain, explicitly detailing its evolutionary necessity.

This is not the case. Not only is this a problem of finding exact emotional fingerprints within the body and brain but it's also a linguistic problem, for the language we use to describe emotion not only influences and frames our experience, but it also limits our personal and cultural understanding of an extremely complex phenomenon.

There are two people who a made significant contribution to the study of emotion back in the 1950s and 1960s and who changed our collective take on these assumptions. The first is the psychologist John Bowlby, who developed attachment theory. Mainstream psychology has come to rely heavily on attachment theory, which states that our emotional behavior is rooted in the primary mother-child relationship we have as an infant. This theory helped lift us out of Victorian-era childrearing and gave credence to the very natural instinct to attend to our child when there's distress. Before this time, raising a child tended to involve severe discipline, letting babies cry it out, and teaching kids to master their emotions through sheer willpower, or if that fails, corporal punishment. In the West, our emotional legacy is one of extreme repression, the consequences of which are still in play today. Attachment theory also bolsters the idea that whereas primitive emotions are instinctive, the pro-social emotions need to be cultivated and taught by proper childrearing.

The second person is psychologist Paul Ekman, whose experiments with tribal peoples untouched by Western culture apparently proved they could successfully identify seven key emotions from pictures of faces shown to them. This established the mainstream acceptance that there are indeed universal emotions with universal facial expressions, an idea with which Darwin would be delighted.

However, the severe emotions of sadness, anger, rage, fear, surprise, happiness, and grief were specifically picked out because in the West we have culturally established facial expressions that reflect these emotions. Before the experiments took place, each subject was vetted so that they could understand what specific emotions were of interest which happened to be the seven emotions highlighted by European culture. Although Ekman's work led to a bulk of research replicating his studies that built on the assumption of universal emotions, they also replicated the intrinsic problems with the methodology.[5] There is significant counterevidence that shows that the same tribal groups do not recognize and categorize emotions in the same way as Western culture.

Ekman went on to develop the Facial Action Coding System, which maps the specific facial muscles that engage with each emotion. Although his work is fascinating and has greatly helped our understanding of how we communicate emotions as a culture, it does not account for the full complexity of emotion. There may indeed be a degree of validity in particular Western social contexts, but even in the West there are many people who express the emotions of fear or anger in atypical ways, just as there are many cultures that have entirely different concepts of emotion. This problem is extremely relevant if we consider facial recognition software and mass surveillance, for we may be inadvertently programming our technologies with false models of emotional expression. Nevertheless, Ekman's work set a precedent that built upon Darwin's evolutionary theory of emotion.

Over the past sixty years the field of neuroscience has made leaps and bounds in unveiling the dizzying complexity of the brain. Neuroscience presented us with the first tool to measure what's happening in the brain, therefore bringing the study of emotion proper scientific validity. Initial steps in this endeavor labeled our more primitive aspects of the brain as the emotional brain and then sought to label the right hemisphere as emotional and the left hemisphere rational and intelligent.

This has led to the popularization of these notions, which have filtered down into psychiatry, psychotherapy, and pop-psychology. For instance, it's popularly known now that the amygdala is the fear center of the brain, cortisol is the neurotransmitter of stress, oxytocin is the neurotransmitter of love, and serotonin equals happiness. However, all of this is simply not true. The brain really is more complex than most people can imagine, and it does not unveil its secrets lightly.

In the same way that we have not found a neural correlate of consciousness, the connections among specific brain regions, pathways, and emotion only describe correlations. They do not give the whole picture; as it turns out, singular emotions can activate many other pathways and regions at the same time. Fear can be experienced without activation of the amygdala, and cortisol can be released without the emotional release of stress or fear.[6] Since the turn of the twenty-first century, neuroscience has been advancing at incredible speed, and the notions that were developed in the 1980s and 1990s have been overturned by new research.

The neuroscientists Joseph LeDoux and Antonio Damasio are two significant researchers who have completely revised our understanding of emotion and the brain. Their work has shown that emotion is not separate from cognition, which means there is no dividing line between cold reason and hot emotion. There is great nuance present in the felt experience of emotion; it is tightly bound to all modes of thinking, perception, and embodiment. This has grave implications for the historical prejudice that civilized humans are rational creatures who can make decisions and form beliefs without the animalistic influence of emotion. If we look to many other cultures, we see thinking and feeling are not always distinct from each other. In classical Chinese philosophy, for instance, thought is classified as a type of emotion.

The pioneer whose research really pronounces a paradigm shift is Lisa Feldman Barrett. Her work homed in on the gaps and anomalies present in Western orthodox thinking about emotion. Specifically, she has highlighted the cultural bias inherent in Darwin's thinking that categorizes emotions into societal norms. Emotions are more easily analyzed when we box them into these seven universal categories, but this limits our understanding of the actual processes behind emotion. It should be reiterated that it's only recently that we have had an objective way to study emotion in the brain. Her research refutes the idea that there are universal pathways in the brain that correspond to each emotion. In other words, there is no biological essence or fingerprint of fear, joy, or anger. Instead, her research shows how emotions are spontaneously constructed in situ (through our living interaction with the world).

Just like we have our own beliefs and habits of posture and language, emotions are gradually learned through childhood. They are not hardwired into us but are live-wired in real time. In particular, we learn emotion from mimicking our parents and caregivers as babies and children. This means emotions are more complex than we previously assumed; they are highly personal in both their outward expression and internal mechanics.

The idea that all humans share universal instinctual facial expressions is too simplistic. We have social and cultural norms, but facial expression varies greatly between both cultures and individuals. Just think of the contrast in how emotions are expressed in Japanese, Russian, Maori, and English cultures. The complexity, subtlety, and mystery of emotion is apparent in others' faces. Because we learn emotion through social interaction and mimicry, the mimic muscles of the face are therefore essential for our ability to relate to others and conceive of emotions internally.

Barrett's theory of socially constructed emotion is a major achievement. It strips away the simplistic idea that emotions are linear instinctual mechanisms and shows instead that our experience of emotion is a highly complex relational process. This relationality of emotion dovetails with Porges's polyvagal theory and Welch and Ludwig's emotional connection theory.* Each of these ways of understanding emotion describes how we are continually regulating one another's nervous systems and emotions through social interaction, through our faces and voices.

There is a continual dance between self-regulation and co-regulation. We are entangled in one another's inner worlds much more than most

---

*Both of these theories are part of a broader expansion of evolutionary theory that explores the relational mechanisms between different organisms, such as the concept of the holobiome. For more info, see Ludwig and Welch, "Darwin's Other Dilemmas and the Theoretical Roots of Emotional Connection."

realize. Practically speaking, this means spending time with people who are calm and lovely will in turn create the feeling of calmness and loveliness in us. Conversely, spending time with people who are stressed and fearful will cue our nervous systems into a stress and fear state. Instead of seeing emotion as one size fits all, this new paradigm of emotion points toward everyone existing in nuanced, emotional worlds, within different spectrums and ranges of feeling.

For instance, whereas one person says he's feeling stressed, another person can clearly differentiate within that feeling of stress a more nuanced mixture of anxiety, depression, or grief. This is called emotional granularity and describes how one person can have a low-resolution spectrum of feeling whereas another person can have a much higher definition, effectively feeling more nuance in their experience of the world.

So, within the feeling of anxiety there might be a whole range of different types of anxiety, some tinged with nostalgia, fear, anger, or even love. Largely, what we call emotional intelligence hinges on our ability to discern what we're feeling with clearer and more nuanced resolution. This, in turn, is significantly shaped by our language.

If we have only one word for love, our capacity for expressing this emotion tends to be limited, which can have the tendency of boxing in what we believe is possible to feel and express toward others. For instance, in ancient Greece there are eight words for love, which differentiate between feelings such as romantic love, brotherly love, and universal love. By contrast, an argument could be made that because our culture has only one word for a whole spectrum of experience, this has contributed to limiting the social acceptability of these more nuanced expressions, a resounding justification for the essential need for increasing our vocabulary, eloquence, and poetry in our everyday speech. Echoing the words of the poet David Whyte, "We can inhabit different words and phrases in a way that opens us to different worlds."

However, a significant key that Barrett's work has revealed for us is how emotion stems largely from interoception, which is our felt sense of what's happening inside our body. This is largely enabled through the vagus nerve, which conveys information about the state of our digestion, muscles, bladder, heart, and so on. Our body senses and communicates important signals to our brain about our health. We tend to think of our senses as only communicating external information, but we also have internal senses that are vitally important.

These physiological signals play a major part in the formation of our emotions. Anyone who's experienced the feeling of being "hangry" knows how easy it is to misinterpret anger with hunger. When we feel our heart racing, we can interpret this either as "I'm having a panic attack" or "I've drunk way too much coffee." And so, it's this felt ability to accurately predict and give meaning to these signals that is crucial to emotional intelligence.

So much of our world is a result of the brain's prediction and interpretation. The feeling of impending doom can be interpreted as either an insignificant emotion or as an early symptom of a heart attack or seizure. And so, our capacity for listening and attuning to our internal sensations should therefore not be derided only as vague intuition but as an important touchstone for health and well-being.

This is where the new science of emotion starts to parallel the much older intuitions that informed indigenous thinking, Chinese medicine, and Dien Chan. On a pragmatic level, this points toward emotional well-being not as something that we can think or talk our way into but as something that must be felt and embodied.

Our whole body is engaged with emotion, not just our brain, head, or face. We are all capable of intuitively appreciating this, for it is quite clear that our heart and gut feelings have a fundamental part to play in our emotional experience. Emotions stem from the relationship between our body and brain; hence, if we can deeply familiarize ourselves with all the nuance and sensation within our bodies and learn to make friends with our nervous system, then this will build the ground for emotional balance. Meeting the body and coming home to the body are therefore essential for healing the negative emotional patterns of stress and trauma.

Before we look at how emotions are understood from the perspective of Dien Chan and Chinese medicine, let us pause and learn a few simple, practical techniques to quickly release tension from our face and mind-body.

NINE

. . . .

Making Faces

We now have an inkling that our faces can become stuck in emotional patterns and masks. Like falling into a groove, we may raise an eyebrow, furrow a brow, or purse our lips entirely without thinking. These habits go on to form the grooves and wrinkles that appear as we age. A useful way to make a pattern-interrupt is to consciously explore the full range of our facial expression. Sometimes this is called face yoga or facial exercise. Such exercises are familiar to professional singers and actors, but they also have therapeutic value if we consider the social nervous system that underwrites our emotional expression. These exercises can be performed in several ways. The following sequence draws from the qigong exercise known as the Horse's Mouth.

❀ The Horse's Mouth: Protocol for Shaking Out and Refreshing the Face

1. Open the eyes wide and lift the eyebrows as far as you can. Open the mouth and jaw as much as you can. Then squeeze the eyes, nose, and mouth together tightly. Repeat this opening and closing of the face, making circular movements, engaging the nose and ears, and exploring the face's full range of movement.

2. Take a big breath in, opening the face. As you exhale, completely

relax the face while blowing air out of the cheeks and lips, like you're imitating a horse. As you exhale, gently release the head forward, like you're dead-weighting the head. Repeat a couple times.

3. Rub and warm the palms together, then vigorously rub and dry-wash the face, sweeping off any tension from the brows and cheeks, then down the ears and neck. (Be careful if you're wearing any jewelry.)

This sequence can be performed very quickly, within thirty seconds, but can have powerful effect. It can be used for a quick reset of our emotional template and as a way to come home to and ground the body.

❧ Three Calming Points

These three Dien Chan points can be used reliably to settle the mind, down-regulate the nervous system, and calm the heart. This sequence is frequently used at the beginning of Dien Chan treatments and is easy to perform as a self-care massage. While these points can be stimulated with a massage tool for a stronger effect, because of their location on the forehead we can elicit a similarly positive response by using our knuckles. For the first two points we bring the hands into loose fists and use the middle knuckle of the index fingers to press the points.

1. Make loose fists and use the middle knuckle of the index fingers to press and slowly sweep horizontally across point 124 (see figure 9.1). This point is located at the halfway line between the eyebrows and the hairline, directly above the outer edges of the iris. You don't need pinpoint accuracy but rather want to make sure you sweep slowly over the point, anywhere from a centimeter to a few inches across the midline of the forehead. See if you can feel your knuckles pass over a little bump toward the sides of the forehead. Make a minimum of three sweeps, or you can slowly press and sweep ten to twenty times according to your needs.

2. With loose fists, hook the index finger around the tip of the thumb so

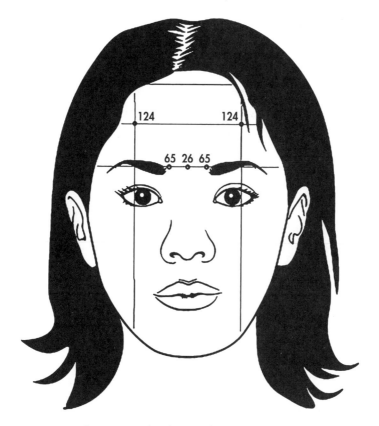

Figure 9.1. The three calming Dien Chan
points—124, 65, and 26

that the knuckles can be used in a more compact way. Slowly press and circle point 65, which is located a few millimeters inside and above the inner corner of the eyebrows. You are pressing in and around the infraorbital foramen, which is a little notch on the bony ridge above the inside corner of the eye. This is where a branch of the trigeminal nerve passes, and so this point can often feel quite sensitive. Because of this, start by pressing lightly and increase to medium pressure, keeping within your comfort zone. Press and circle for a minimum of five to ten seconds.

3. With the left hand, use the tip of the middle finger to press point 26, also known as the third-eye point, or the *Yin Tang*/Hall of Spirit point, and

located at the center of the brow, midway between the two 65 points. Instead of using normal pressure, begin by simply hovering the fingertip a few millimeters away from the point, then, with as slow and light a touch as possible, make contact with the point. Increase the pressure only minimally, and then release your hand. It can be helpful to do this with the eyes closed, but do what feels good for you.

There are two other good options for working with this point. The first is to use the same fingertip to tap very lightly, up to one hundred times. Make sure to tap only with the muscles and energy of the finger and wrist, so the shoulder and elbow remain relatively relaxed. This alternative technique can also be used by itself to help get to sleep. The second option is to use the knuckle to press and slowly sweep upward over the point, which gives a stronger release and tends to have a more focusing rather than calming quality.

TEN

Emotions in Dien Chan & Chinese Medicine

Life is a vortex of water—a whirlpool. Or a flame. Change is part of its very being.

J. B. S. HALDANE

The external form of the stream is stable only because of the constant flow of water molecules that enter into it and emerge out of it.

LUDWIG VON BERTALANFFY

When trying to understand how Chinese medicine has traditionally viewed emotions we must resist the oversimplification that is apparent in the modern popularizations of this tradition. If we hear that fear is a product of the kidneys, or anger an expression of the liver, this obscures the full artistry of this healing modality.

In reality, the views of Chinese medicine practitioners have always been diverse and pluralistic and have always reflected the cultural, geographic, and historical changes that have occurred over the past three thousand years. There is no single correct representation of Chinese medicine. Within Chinese, Vietnamese, Japanese, Korean, and Western acupuncture there have been many different ideas and approaches to emotion and embodiment. Nevertheless, among this great variety of opinion there has always been a respect and deference to the original tenets of the tradition, which are laid out in the classical text known as the *Nei Jing Su Wen (The Yellow Emperor's Inner Classic)*.* In this ancient tome we find a similarity to the notion that emotions arise via interoception; they stem from our physical body.

However, the original authors went further and stated that specific organs were connected to and in resonance with specific emotional processes. For instance, in chapter 23 we read:

> When the heart is overly abundant, symptoms such as hysteria or giggling will manifest; when the lung is overly abundant, grief and crying will manifest; when the liver is overly abundant, it overacts on the spleen and there is an excess of worrying; when the spleen is overly abundant, it overacts on the kidneys and there is a tendency toward being timid.[1]

If we interpret this paragraph without the nuance of a symbolic viewpoint, we might assume that all grief is due to what's happening in our lungs. This is, of course, incorrect. If we look to the last two sentences, we see how there is a relationality among the organs, which then manifests in emotion. If we look further on in the chapter, we see that this relationality is also happening between each organ and its embeddedment within an ecology of pathogens—"When the pathogen travels from the yang level to the yin, the symptoms will quiet down, and the patient will become withdrawn. When the illness

---

*It should be noted that the *Nei Jing Su Wen* was in turn highly influenced and reliant on the Dao De Jing, Yi Jing, and the Yin Yang school of thought. Being able to correctly interpret the Nei Jing Su Wen depends on being well versed in these slightly older philosophical classics. This illustrates the interconnection between medicine and philosophy in ancient China.

travels from yin to yang, the patient will have outbursts of anger."[2]

Considering that this text is more than two thousand years old, it's remarkable that it describes how our emotional behavior is in dialogue with environmental pathogens, something that modern virology has only started to discover in recent decades. Chinese medicine tracks the various ways that our organs and internal physiology reflects our emotional expression and how this process can manifest in disease. From this more complex viewpoint, we can see that our different organs are in resonance with a multitude of emotions, as well as what are called virtues—such as compassion, wisdom, and integrity.

This entanglement between the health of our organs and our emotional expression is seen as a primary concern for overall well-being and healing. Both Chinese medicine and modern neuroscience tell us that emotions are not disconnected from the physical systems of the body; they are interwoven through our hormonal system, microbiome, bones, brain, and nervous system. Because Chinese medicine has traditionally held a more integrated conception of mind and body, our emotional lives have held a central place in both disease and healing. The implication of this means that the way in which we respond to the trials and turbulence of life directly affects our physical health.

However, over the centuries and millennia different theories, approaches, and therapeutics have emerged regarding how to best harmonize our emotions. This variety of opinion reflects the changes in culture, local geography, climate, religion, and the politics of the time. This means there is no absolute consensus, and some doctors take an essentialist perspective that views specific emotions as only pertaining to specific organs, whereas others see emotions in a more complex, fluid, and dynamic way.*

---

*This debate is still fully alive within the five element theory, or Worseley school of acupuncture, which tends to see people as being born into a constitutional element and therefore being fixed into emotional dynamics. Many practitioners, both historically and currently, employ the theory of five elements without the overly fixed or essentialist perspective.

This plurality of opinion might be seen as a weakness but is actually a concealed strength, for it keeps our learning process open-ended rather than in a closed loop of certainty. This is particularly important for the many complex health issues that pertain to the spirit. When our perspective is open-ended, we can see another person or situation from multiple, different vantage points, giving us a flexibility that allows us to adapt to each individual circumstance rather than apply a cookie-cutter protocol for everyone. This flexibility is part of the blueprint of Chinese medicine, which can arguably be traced to the foundational text of Chinese civilization, the Yi Jing. It's said that in each statement of the Yi Jing the opposite can also be inferred. Like a Zen koan, this breaks the rigidity of habituated thinking patterns.

In Chinese medicine this flexibility is not only an intellectual skill that helps diagnosis but also is an embodied skill that is quite different from modern medical practice. Most Western doctors try to remain emotionally aloof, maintaining as much as possible a perspectival knowing that is based purely on what is objective. Chinese medicine doctors engage a participatory knowing, one that is interactive with both the physicality of each client and also attuned to the mental-emotional dynamics. The doctor's subjective emotional feedback is of great value.* So long as there is a keen receptivity within the doctor, the emotional resonance of the heart offers diagnostic insight into the interiority of the patient.

The reason why Chinese medicine is so reliant on this flexibility of perspective is based on a foundational idea at the heart of Chinese philosophy and culture. This idea is deceptively simple: everything changes. How we respond to the changing circumstance of life dictates the course of our lives. It's nearly too obvious to state, but this

---

*Many practitioners take it further and consider the participation, dialogue, and emotional connection to each client as therapeutic in and of itself—the doctor is the medicine. This has some similarity to the Western branch of psychotherapy known as relational therapy, which would rephrase it as, "relationship is the medicine".

idea is readily and consistently forgotten when it comes to our emotional lives.

Instead, we often inhabit emotions as the unchanging house of our being. This solidifying of emotion over time shapes our character and temperament. And when emotion becomes too fixed, it starts to constrain and inhibit our health, an idea that is quite generally accepted throughout the healing traditions of East Asia, as it seems to be a universal aspect of human growth. To grow into an adult or an elder we need to disinhibit ourselves from the emotional templates we form in the earlier stages of our life.

This dynamic between being fixed and changing/growing is descriptive of good health in general: anything that does not change is liable to become diseased. This can be seen most readily in the heartbeat, blood flow, and movement of breath. If these stop flowing and changing, we die. If a cell stops changing, it becomes a cancerous tumor. If an emotion stops changing, we call it mental illness. In simple terms, illness is that which does not change. This is summed up in the adage Tong Ze Bu Tong, to Bu Tong Ze Tong, which translates to, "If there is free flow, there is no pain; if there is pain, there is lack of free flow."

This same idea refers to both physical and emotional pain. The sense of being stuck and stagnant can be released by increasing circulation to the mind-body. In this case, the right type of body movement and exercise is a key therapeutic tool for healing both physical and emotional pain. This is the same primary principle for healing in all types of massage, reflexology, and acupuncture: disinhibit the body of contraction, poor circulation, and stagnation. It's also supported by the evidence that exercise and movement are key to healing both pain and depression.[3]

However, this does not address the question of how we should respond in the more immediate experience of emotion. Movement, massage, and exercise help in the wake of emotional turmoil, but how do we remain free, spontaneous, and open in the immediacy of the moment?

It is not so simple as just going for a walk, although this is not always the worst idea. How do we free ourselves from the deeply ingrained emotional patterns and psychosclerosis of the mind? A cold glare will rapidly contract our mind, just as a cold wind will contract our blood vessels.

This is where different schools of thought diverge, as there is a great subtlety and nuance between how emotions are personally experienced, how they are socially perceived, and how they are intellectually understood. We all wear emotional masks to deceive other people of our own emotions, whether to help ease and soothe other peoples' feelings or to bolster our self-image. We all have various poker faces that help us play the social status games of society.

It's sometimes suggested that people are only capable of emotional openness and vulnerability within the confines of intimate friendship and privacy and that we inherently put on brave faces in all public situations. In all cultures there are various degrees of "saving face," of behaving in ways that comply with social norms and avoid unnecessary embarrassment. But, even outside of public situations, within the privacy of our close kinships, or even when we are completely alone, we also put on masks. We have an incredible capacity for self-deception, which can disconnect us from the deeper implications of our emotions. The layers of masks that constitute our identity beg the question: What is my authentic self behind all the masks? What is my original face?

In Chinese culture, the traditional ways of understanding emotion stem largely from the three main religions: Daoism, Confucianism, and Buddhism. These three religions all have philosophical guidance for how we should behave toward one another and how to best manage our personal experience of emotion. The study of emotion in Chinese medicine can't be separated from these philosophical and spiritual beliefs.

At its heart, Chinese medicine is rooted in the Daoist worldview. Within Daoism there is an aspiration to be like water, to flow naturally in accordance with life's changes.[4] This way of being is called *wei wu wei,* which translates variously as "action without action" or "effortlessness." It hinges on the belief that if we can live our life in harmony with the ever-flowing patterns of change in nature, then good health and spiritual harmony will arise.

Wei wu wei is often described as a state of being that is both natural and spontaneous. Historically, this is where opinions have clashed, because although Chinese culture has its deepest roots in Daoism, the separate tradition of Confucianism offered alternative models for being in harmony with nature. Whereas Daoism is perhaps addressed more to our personal behavior as an individual, Confucianism explicitly concerns the affairs of society and governance and lays out a strict code for how families and communities should behave.

This is where some disagreement comes in, as the virtues of an individual person do not necessarily apply in the same way to large-scale society. Although these two philosophical viewpoints both agreed on cultivating harmony with nature, Confucianism systematized the patterns of nature into a hierarchical blueprint for how families, businesses, and governments should be organized. Central to this notion is the emotion called Xiao, or filial piety, a type of love and respect for one's parents, which was also extended to one's elders and superiors in society. The virtue we cultivate as people is thus an essential ingredient in societal harmony and, on a deeper level, is reflective of an inherent virtue within the natural world.

Daoists have poked fun at this idea because the more superior someone becomes in society, the more likely they will lose their virtue and connection to nature. As is often said, power corrupts; hence, we shouldn't enforce our expectations too rigidly on other people but instead adapt to each relationship with good humor and flexibility. The emotional dynamics surrounding social status and the juxtaposition between the individual and the community are the big issues with which Daoism and Confucianism contend. This is a simplified explanation of an extremely complex history, akin to trying to explain Christianity and Judaism in a few sentences.[5]

Approximately one thousand years after the early formation of Daoism and Confucianism, a third religion was embraced by Chinese culture—Buddhism. It is these three religions that formed the basis for how emotions were handled and thought about in both culture and medicine. Although they present different angles on the specifics of emotion and what is correct behavior, over time they were largely integrated together. As the saying goes, "The Chinese gentleman wears a Confucian hat, Daoist robes, and Buddhist sandals."*

This situation added to the diversity in perspective we see in Chinese medicine and how opinions shifted from century to century in accordance with the prominence and changes to each religion. Whereas Buddhism tends to offer a more systematic exploration into the nature of the mind, Confucianism offered guidance for social relationships and Daoism for our relationship with nature. All three, therefore, have relevance for understanding our emotional expression and how to conduct ourselves in a way that optimizes health and social well-being. A common thread shared between all, and in fact shared in most spiritual practices, is an emphasis on the cultivation of virtue.

Specifically, virtue is framed as an innate human quality that compels us to act with empathy, compassion, and kindness to others. In the West, virtue is often framed side-by-side with the notion of original sin and, therefore, as something that we inherently lack and need to redeem in ourselves. In modern times it is framed as entirely socially constructed, without any biological basis.

In the East, virtue is more readily framed as intrinsic to human nature. A newly born baby has an innate type of virtue, which is termed the heart of the Dao. It is only through living that it is obscured by the suffering of trauma and the inevitable entanglement

---

*Notice the implications for how these traditions relate to our embodiment.

in worldly deceptions and desires. Although this might seem like a small point, it's quite fundamental to how we treat other humans and our own self-relationship. It comes back to the veneer theory of human emotion—that if we scratch the surface of our apparent civility, what is revealed is a ruthless drive for self-survival. This is often summed up by the adage of any decent person being only three meals away from barbarity.* Whether we see our human behavior as fundamentally rooted in kindness or rooted in selfishness reflects how we approach life: Is the world intrinsically a place of hostility and malevolence? Or is the heart of the world benevolent? Or simply a place of uncaring indifference?

If we reframe ourselves as fundamentally kindhearted beings, this makes a powerful step toward engendering greater self-love and self-compassion, which in turn strengthens our capacity for love and forgiveness in all our relations. This attitude is common in both Daoism, Confucianism, and Buddhism. In Buddhism, it is expressed in the term Bodhicitta, or Buddha Mind, which describes all of reality as sharing in the enlightened state, and which is the undercurrent to human virtue.

In Daoism, the source text is titled Dao De Jing, which is translated as "The Way and its Virtue." Implicit in the title is that the Way imbues life with virtue, one that is expressed in both the natural world and human nature. In Confucianism, virtue is the keystone to all relationship. But, at the grandest scale, Confucianism connects the virtue of nature specifically to the Chinese emperor, similar to what in medieval times was called the divine right of kings. This shows how there is some overlap, as well as variance, with the Eastern conception of virtue, and that it's also quite different from traditional Western notions and language.

In both the East and West, virtue can easily fall into societally defined norms, which can easily make people skeptical of all systems of morality or susceptible to a kind of cynicism, apathy, and nihilism.

---

*Coincidently, this is the maxim for the British Intelligence Service, MI5.

However, what many religious and spiritual traditions point toward is a hidden thread that weaves together our biology, sociality, and spirituality. In other words, virtue is not purely a social construct or culturally relative. Nor is nature fundamentally without virtue.

Our modern culture has a large blind spot surrounding this issue, one that lies just beyond the horizon of the reasoning and empirical mind. And even though it is difficult to intellectually grasp beyond this horizon, we nevertheless have an imaginative faculty that can sense in to this unknown terrain. This is the aforementioned mythical sensibility, our capacity to contend with multiple orders of truth. Instead of seeing things purely as a binary of good and evil, we can frame virtue as a complex and multivalent way of orienting toward others. The sages and seers who've developed this faculty report that underneath all the social fabrications and the genetic explanations of morality, there is a principle and pattern within our being and nature that expresses unconditional compassion, love, and kindness.

For some people this makes perfect sense; love is the strongest impulse in the world. For others, there is a visceral repulsion to this idea, as if it's the height of wishful thinking and stupidity—a clear failure of critical thinking. The ability to change our scale of thinking will determine where we stand on this. At one end there is a unitive and collaborative vision of harmony, at the other end an eventual relinquishment to nothingness and nihilism. We must recognize that nature is chock full of the most profound suffering and agony. But instead of writing off the notion of universal love, can we entertain the possibility that life is much grander and more complex than we might imagine? Can we sustain the query of "What if?"

To feel into this complexity is to shift from what the education specialist Zachary Stein calls a pre-tragic to a post-tragic mode of being. He argues that for many people, and for culture-at-large, we get stuck in a cycle between a pre-tragic naïveté and the trauma of life's tragedies, without ever finding a true resolution.[6] When we only see suffering and life as a battle for survival, this takes us down a destructive spiral. As the mythologist Martin Shaw once said, "If you only look into hell, eventually you turn to ashes."

If we only take the natural world to be hostile, amoral, and poisonous, we miss the outrageous generosity, beauty, and medicine that nature provides. But if we can break the cycle and draw from nature's impulse to regenerate and renew itself, despite wanton destruction, we might reach a grander and more majestic vision of our lives, one that's infused with vivid potential, creativity, and awe. This is akin to the post-tragic stance that can draw sustenance and resilience from the suffering of life.

Whether or not we place any stock in these ideas, at a more immediate and personal level, virtue does not have to be some lofty ideal or mystical property but can simply be a willingness to listen and remain open to possibility. In itself, our capacity to listen to others and our body is a form of kindness. It's an aspirational stance, for it is seeking out a positive mutual outcome. It's the opposite of closing off and fighting with our bodies or closing our ears to others. In response to the conniving mind that might argue people only listen to others so they might gain advantage from them, I would expand our definition of *listening* using listening expert Alan Alda's words: "True listening is the willingness to be changed by the other person."[7]

In this sense, virtue isn't so much something one has but is more akin to a compass that can be oriented toward it. This orientation happens both socially, with our faces and voices, and internally, in our body, heart, and mind. Listening to this compass is similar to being mindful and open to the unfolding presence of what is, being able to stay with the trouble rather than dissociating or burying one's head in the sand. What the old traditions suggest is that this compass is not mine, it's not personal, but is rather encompassed through our relationality. In other words, virtue arises in the dialogue between beings rather than being possessed by one or the other.

And so, this brings us back to the unusual notion of effortless action, wei wu wei, for it's this stance that is said to attune us to the natural and optimal approach of emotional expression. This attunement connects us with the inherent virtue in nature. This is the same virtue that powers the body's natural ability for regeneration and healing. Emotionally, this attunement affords us harmony and coherence between our social lives and the emotions that flow through us. We can respond in ways that are not detrimental to ourselves or others and are at the same time appropriate to any given circumstance, an ideal much easier said than done. As Aristotle once noted in his classic work *The Art of Rhetoric*: Anybody can become angry—that is easy, but to be angry with the right person and to the right degree and at the right time and for the right purpose, and in the right way—that is not within everybody's power and is not easy."

Although there are multiple interpretations of what is involved in wei wu wei, to my own understanding it's a type of deep listening to the moment-to-moment change that is occurring both inside and outside the mind-body. It's a somatic skill just as much an orientation of thought. It's not simply going with the flow and letting emotions run wild. Rather, it is a willingness to remain open and refrain from absolute certainty. This willingness to remain in uncertainty is closely akin to keeping in touch with the felt body.

What this points toward is that our embodiment is a crucial aspect of emotional health and can be described in Daoist fashion as inner listening or interoception and vagal tone. More specifically, there is a directionality to our embodiment that can either impede the flow of emotions or digest and integrate them. When we close off to our bodies this has the effect of contracting our world into fixed certainties. This in turn makes emotion tighten or linger inside of us. Often this is expressed as a physical tightening of the face, where our awareness and energy is clenched into the head. But when we embrace the flowing of the world through us, this helps integrate emotions so we don't become stuck in loops, patterns, and contractions in our mind-body.

What both the Golden Elixir practices and Dien Chan reveal is that the direction of integration is earthbound—there is a downward flow from our face, down to our heart and belly. Notice that when we make a deep sigh of relief, the motion is one of releasing the face and chest, as if we are unburdening and emptying our hearts of any strain. When we open to this downward flow, which is a matter of coming deeper and deeper in touch with our vagal pathway, we can seamlessly integrate not only our present experience but also transform undigested emotions and experiences from our past.

An insight I've realized from my personal practice of Dien Chan and meditation is that the subtle tension held in the face inhibits us from fully inhabiting our body and from being able to settle our awareness downward into the body. This kind of facial tension is normally under the radar of our conscious experience, but when we reach progressively more and more relaxed and clear states of consciousness in meditation, the tension held in the face can suddenly become apparent, and when we release the facial tension, we find ourselves entering more profound states of stillness and concentration. Dien Chan and the self-care massage techniques of the Golden Elixir make this process much easier. They open the pathways of release between the head and body as well as between the greater fields of energy that surround our body.

A helpful image to use is that of a whirlpool. In many river bends and streams you might notice small whirlpools that retain their form due to the dynamic among rock, riverbed, and water. Although they have a constant stream of water passing through them, their form remains stable due to this continuous inflow. This is like our mind-body.* We

---

*I am indebted to Philip Shepherd for the image of the body as whirlpool, which in turn is echoed in the words of J. B. S. Haldane and Alfred North Whitehead.

digest all experience, emotional or otherwise, through our embodiment. Our body and mind are constantly changing but will remain stable and healthy so long as we keep the inflow of our experience flowing through us and don't take on more than we can bear, like the whirlpool taking on sediment or, in our case, becoming overly embroiled in emotion. When emotion suffuses every moment of our lives, our experience of newness and freshness is gradually blocked. We become existentially stuck, and it's this state that becomes harmful for our health.

Notice that this image doesn't suggest we shouldn't experience or express emotion. This would be equally as detrimental, for it would halt the inflow of new experience. In terms of our embodiment, this means learning to frame our physical and mental posture in a way that is both constantly welcoming in, while continuously letting go. It's like an optimal grip, held not too tight, or too soft. This allows us to adapt and respond to each situation with a natural accordance. A mythical image that describes this poise is a person sitting in a room with two windows. Two birds swoop into the window singing, "I am coming, I am coming." At the same time, two birds fly out of the other window, singing, "I am going, I am going."

The ability to welcome in new experience is closely connected with being able to savor, delight in, and feel wonder. The ability to let go is closely connected with equanimity but also opens us to humor, lightheartedness, and forgiveness. Equanimity is a mind-body state that can remain neutral to experience—neither grasping nor pushing away. It's an ability to sit within the fire of our experience without flinching, to tolerate the harshness of the world.

Equanimity is a deep background quality of our mind that allows our body to physically relax. The relaxation of our muscles and nervous system happens in stages, deepens through gradations. Being relaxed is not something that's ever complete—we discover there are always deeper states of relaxation. This is the remarkable skill that meditation develops, and if we simply keep letting go and relaxing further and further, equanimity can reveal states of bliss and rapture in the deep background of our normal, everyday experience.

When we press a point on the face or body and it's tender, equanimity allows us to release into the tenderness and not flinch or contract against the pressure. This quality of mind plays a key role both in healing and developing wisdom. The downward flow of energy releases us into the felt sense of the body and also brings us in touch with our inherent body wisdom, toward a more vivid and direct encounter with ourselves and the nature of consciousness.

If we consider how both Buddhists and neuroscientists understand the nitty-gritty formation of emotion, there is a clear parallel. Neuroscientists break emotion down into what is known as affect, which is thought to be the psychosomatic precursor and building block of emotion. Affect is categorized into three basic responses: pleasure, displeasure, and indifference. Likewise, Buddhist doctrine understands that emotions derive from three basic responses: desire, aversion, and ignorance.

The word *ignorance* implies both a confusion toward the nature of life and also a lack of awareness—like a checking out from experience. It's different from the state of unknowing, which is so positive for creativity and humility. We can see ignorance has an overlap with the affect category of indifference. However, I believe within the understanding of this affect category, the mental quality of equanimity has gone under the radar, because there is a very fine and subtle distinction between how the brain appears when it's indifferent and how we feel when we are equanimous. Equanimity has an openness of attention that is lacking in indifference.

Equanimity has profound implications for the moment-to-moment creation of our conscious mind and the disentanglement of emotional patterns. Therefore, equanimity is regarded as the key to liberating the mind in Buddhist Vipassana meditation. Regardless, equanimity is a natural mind-body state to which we all have access, just like we all have the ability to consciously relax our breathing and our bodies. The phrase "it is what it is" helps us accept the present moment and not fight or tense up against our present reality. The downward flow describes the natural way we ground ourselves, integrate emotion, and shift into deeper states of calmness and equanimity.

There are two aspects to this downward flow that are worth unpacking. The first is that the current of the whirlpool needs to flow down continuously—we need a sustained ability to feel in to our bodies if we are to affect vagal tone. Most people have a common tendency for awareness to jump back up into our heads and senses. This in turn is associated with a tightening of the shoulders, chest, breath, and face. Inversely, releasing physical or emotional tension from the face creates a downward cascade into the body, helping ground us and bringing stability to the mind-body. When this happens in a sustained flow, it changes and transforms the patterns in our nervous system and embodiment. We feel calm, safe, and at home in the world, which allows for the real-time integration of old emotion and trauma.

Second, we need to consider what we are flowing down toward. Some people don't give enough credit to the power of interoception and might say they have zero awareness of any organs of the body, and if it wasn't for people telling them, they'd have no clue about their liver or kidneys! This actually reflects their reality, as the trauma specialist Steve Haines says, "One of the biggest insights I have had from clinical experience is that most people are poor at feeling their body."[8] In fact, we have the ability to change how much nuance we feel inside our bodies. This is what developing vagal tone is all about. And the way to do this is to slowly sustain our attention on the felt sense of the body.

The first and most noticeable sensation is usually that of our heart pulsing in our chest. If we can listen to our heartbeat, we may notice the pulsing of blood flow around the body. In meditation, this skill of discerning the felt body is taken to a high art, with the ability to differentiate the organs; the feeling of the skin compared with the bones; the different chambers of the heart; and even into more subtle aspects of the mind-body. It is through this kind of meditation that the insights of Buddhism came about, which revealed the body in greater clarity, as well as the nature of mind and emotion.

One of the key insights both Buddhism and Daoism share, and fundamental to Chinese medicine, is that the human heart plays a vital role in consciousness. The Chinese medical term for the heart is *Xin* and describes both the physical organ and a specific dimension of our consciousness and emotion. This framing of the heart as an organ of consciousness is foundational to Chinese medicine. But rather than thinking of the heart in the same way we think of the brain, we think about how its role in consciousness is like the deep undertone that lies beneath the cognitive workings of the mind. This undertone provides the stability of the mind, which is when the quality of our awareness is clear, still, and calm. There is a clear parallel between vagal tone and the Chinese concept of the Xin, or heart-mind, for the heart is innervated by the vagus nerve, and the vagus nerve is intimately involved in emotional regulation.

The downward flow describes our ability to come to rest in the heart. From an experiential standpoint, this ability to be embodied—to live and speak from the heart—changes how we move and behave. In the meditative traditions, heart consciousness reveals the nature of our mind, both personally and universally, because in the Buddhist and Daoist understanding, the deepest background to our heart awareness (our heart of hearts) is a state of natural consciousness that is entirely void of personal ownership. It's this aspect of the heart that reflects the inherent virtue of nature. This reflects the emptiness and interdependence that suffuses all reality. It's this hidden, original, and natural quality of consciousness that is called Shen Ming—the luminosity of spirit—which illuminates our inherent blueprint toward wholeness and self-healing. Our heart acts as a conduit for Shen Ming; it can bring us into greater resonance with the empty field of universal awareness. It's for this reason that in Chinese medicine the heart is symbolically named the Sovereign Emperor. It empowers us with true sovereignty, and this power is expressed in our natural ability for self-healing. Therefore, it's said, "all healing comes from the heart."

Often, we might think of sovereignty as being in full possession of ourselves, but the idea of ownership over our domain can quickly turn to tyranny. True sovereignty holds the wisdom of our inter-being, and this involves being in service to what is greater than us. The tyrant does not submit to anyone; the true king is in full sub-mission to the land and people. This submission is embodied person-ally through a deep listening and attunement to our heart and naval center.

The ability to stay connected and in tune with this empty field is both a key aspect of wei wu wei as well as central for optimal health and healing. Although this might give us the impression this field is like some secret meditation technique only privileged masters can access, in reality we can never be disconnected from it—we are always held within this field, no matter how polluted and terrible our state of body, mind, and environment might seem to be. Every night, we dissociate from our bodies, and the healing balm of deep sleep gives us a full, restorative immersion in this field. We are dreamed anew. This reflects how our original nature is inherently of virtue. Our bod-ies' natural inclination toward regeneration, healing, and wholeness is an expression of this virtue. Dien Chan and many contemplative embodiment practices harness this power for both personal and rela-tional healing.

The connection between our heart, face, and our ability to restore, heal, and renew is rooted in embryology—our invisible *coming into* *being* before we were born. The physical tissues of the face and heart are embryologically entwined: in utero, our origination posture (the fetal position) starts from a deep bow of our faces into our hearts. Our face and heart unfurl from an original source of connection. There is an embodied mirroring between these two aspects of our mind-body, and this gives us a subtle remembrance of this original connection. Dien Chan details this mirroring with a map that overlays the image of the heart onto the face, and also a map which overlays the face over the chest. This mirroring is also suggested through polyvagal theory, which shows how the expressivity and orientation of the face directly synchronizes with the heart rate and heart rate variability.* Our heart and face mirror each other and the world around us.

From the traditional perspective, this multidirectional mirroring reflects our interdependence with the world. That we are mirrors of the world means that it's through our heart perception that we *call forth* the world into being. The suggestion is that we are relational creatures not only because humans are hypersocial but also because every aspect of the world is co-arising in relationality. The mirroring is happening within nervous systems, perception, and the world-at-large.

Taking this further, when the face and heart are embodied in a living relationship, this opens up a resonance with the greater field dynamics of Shen Ming, or the principle of natural renewal. This embodied relationship is like a remembrance of our deep embryology and is what Daoist's call the heart of the Dao, which I mentioned earlier. This is an arbiter, not only for physical healing and regeneration, but also for social and ecological harmony. The felt sense of our inward orientation forms a kind of reciprocity with our external sense orientation. This brings us in touch with the living processes and unknown becomings of the world. It means we can listen to other people with an ear to how

---

*See the footnote on page 159 in the following chapter for more information on heart rate variability.

they are changing and growing and not only to how their past has presented them. This immanent relational aspect to healing is important, because our sense of who we are is continuously re-imagined through our interactions with others. Our sense of who we are and what we are capable of is reinforced most strongly by the people we've known longest. And so, emotional healing is a continuous process that is reaffirmed through our interactions with friends, family, and strangers, as well as people we dislike or who wish us ill will.

Whereas, from a modern viewpoint of the physiology of emotion, we could say our nervous systems are continuously recalibrating in response to other people and signs of threat and safety; the viewpoint from the traditional perspective draws upon a different framework of consciousness—it leads to a different stance and orientation to life. This stance can be summed up as radical compassion. Instead of this being a theoretical musing of some kind of perfect attitude toward others, radical compassion stems from people who have directly experienced nontypical states of consciousness and emotion—states that are sometimes labeled unconditional love.

The classic parable of unconditional love is that of the Buddha who's on the road and is by happenstance accompanied by his mother, best friend, and worst enemy. They are approached by a murderous bandit, who gives Buddha the ultimatum—"I am going to kill one of you four, but I will give you the choice of who dies." The decision is deemed impossible, for one with unconditional love honestly can't distinguish between the love held for himself, mother, friend, or enemy. For most people, this is indeed a strange and unusual type of love. Nevertheless, there are many accounts of strange and unusual people who embody this type of consciousness, and it's this phenomenon that frames the more expansive stance to the world. Love is experienced as a more-than-human reciprocity within the world. The great poet Dante described being in a state where

I glowed with a flame of charity which moved me to forgive all who had ever injured me; and if at that moment someone had asked me a question, about anything, my only reply would have been, "Love."[9]

Speaking of the Buddhist practice of metta, or unconditional loving-kindness, the meditation teacher Rob Burbea says:

Such a practice . . . may initially seem quite naive. As understanding develops over time, we see that it is in fact the opposite; and that a belief that others are objectively and simply how they appear to us would, rather, be naive.[10]

Although radical compassion might seem too saintly for some, the underlying rationale stands firm—no person is undeserving of love or compassion. Again, the strength of conviction for this lies in direct experience, not just in thinking and reasoning. Radical compassion is radical precisely because it's unjustified and unreasonable. It's not a ploy to gain favor but instead a spontaneous response that occurs when this state of unconditional love touches otherness.

It is very likely that what is being pointed to here transcends our normal concept of emotion. This is why the traditional Buddhist language for these non-typical states classifies them differently, too—not as emotions but as *sublime abidings*. There are undoubtedly other names for these states within other cultures. In either case, they are closely related to experiencing our true nature—our original face. In other terms, this is called emptiness, Shen Ming, or the heart of the Dao. Krishnamurti described this beautifully when he said, "Compassion is the essence of the wholeness of life."

Many might dismiss these religious-sounding names or scoff at what is outside their personal experience, but this risks missing a vitally important point: this way of being in the world affects both our personal health and what gives meaning to our lives. If we take the opposite position, that the world is a place of utter indifference and is inherently hostile, we might find that the greater questions of meaning and purpose are negated by the framing of nature as purely a violent bloodbath. This blinds us to the possibility that life, in fact, is not in conflict with itself, that nature might actually be a place of fundamental belonging, safety, and acceptance. By extension, our own lives might be imbued with an entirely natural impulse toward generosity, love, and compassion.

This viewpoint is entirely congruous with many of the great sages, poets, and scientists—both within historical Chinese and traditional cultures and up into the modern day. This viewpoint doesn't deny death, cruelty, corruption, or injustice. But it reframes our orientation toward them, so we have the wisdom to aspire toward creativity rather than simply the avoidance of destruction. The post-tragic orientation takes seriously the notion that there is "no sinner without a future." When the theologian and evolutionary theorist Pierre Teilhard de Chardin said, "Love is the affinity which links and draws together the elements of the world. . . Love, in fact, is the agent of universal synthesis,"[11] he wasn't simply speculating—he was speaking from experience.

This is, of course, something beyond the bounds of our current science and what mainstream culture deems acceptable. It's beyond the horizon of analytical thinking. However, I side with the poets on this one. Rabindranath Tagore tells us: "Love is not mere human sentiment but the heart of existence itself." Dante speaks of a "love that moves the sun and the other stars." How we relate to our bodies and the world-at-large moves us toward this grander and more encompassing vision of life, one that gives us a deep, radiant contentment in both inhabiting our body and the natural world around us. This joie de vivre and loving the world despite everything births hope and possibility, giving impetus for our bodies to jump up and live again—to resuscitate from sickness and dismay.

Dien Chan can be an incredible tool to help re-pattern this continual process of coming home to a more natural state of contentment in the body, for it unbinds the fixed emotional habits that constrict our faces and hearts. It opens a window of opportunity to change how we face the world. In the next chapter we'll delve into the methods for unblocking and re-patterning emotional habits with Dien Chan.

ELEVEN

. . . .

Dien Chan
for Emotional Healing

Enter the bowl of vastness that is the heart.
Listen to the song that is always resonating . . .
Again and again, answer that call,
And be saturated with knowing,
I belong here, I am at home.

THE VIJNANA BHAIRAVA TANTRA,
LORIN ROCHE, TRANS.

In Dien Chan there is no emotional map, as it is recognized that the emotional patterns that we hold in our faces are personally nuanced in expression. Your particular expression of grief, dismay, fear, or anger isn't something that can fit into a fixed template, meaning there is unfortunately no magical point on the face that will universally resolve anger issues or make one's grief disappear.

However, Dien Chan nevertheless has incredible potency for emotional healing, because we all have holding patterns in our faces that link directly into our nuanced emotional history. Dien Chan offers us a way to slowly discover and release these holding patterns. And when we release the face, we create a cascade effect of relaxation down into our heart and belly, strengthening our connection with our body and supporting emotional well-being.

When we feel safe and at home in our body, it becomes possible to integrate our emotions and move toward a sense of wholeness. The self-care practices of Dien Chan are therefore particularly apt for rewriting the stories we hold in our faces. By stimulating points and areas of tension on the face, we open a window of possibility to change and reengage with how we feel, express, and metabolize emotion.

Even though there is no emotional map, Dien Chan does provide clues and methods for exploring particular emotions. In Chinese medicine and Dien Chan theory, each organ has a particular resonance within certain ranges of emotion. And so, by stimulating the different areas on the face, which correlate with each organ, we can elicit both a physical and emotional response. When we touch upon a holding pattern—which is sometimes indicated by a tenderness or change in sensitivity—we may actually feel emotion alight with different areas of the face. Just like that good feeling of pain and release in massage, there can be an emotionally equivalent release. To access this, it is particularly helpful to hold an attitude of listening inward and be open and curious. Also, the aforementioned downward flow, which is like a sigh of relief, is the natural pathway for releasing the face.

The facial areas and points that link into specific emotions are one way of working toward emotional balance. We don't always need this degree of specificity, though, as the broader effect of reconnecting our head with our heart lays the groundwork for feeling stronger and more resilient in mind and body.

Massaging the face can be incredibly relaxing and blissful; it can soothe our troubled minds and hearts, bringing us toward increased feelings of safety and calm, which is both the first step in healing and also a type of resourcing that can create much positive change in and of itself. Learning to do this ourselves and realizing we have this power to change our state of being can gradually allow us to change and re-pattern our orientation response. Our face (and physiological state) can stay relaxed and open when we encounter the challenges of the world, rather than immediately default to a stress response.

The downward flow of release follows the pathway of the vagus nerve and allows us to come to rest in the body. By increasing our felt sense of the body, we increase vagal tone, both increasing our sense of calm and presence and enabling us to feel with more depth and texture into our bodies and emotional states. And so, a regular Dien Chan self-care practice can create a positive feedback loop that strengthens our ability to remain calm in the face of adversity and be a light to others. It can help us remain present in a fully embodied way and start to rediscover our bodies in new ways, too.

We all tend to have parts of our body we feel a little disconnected from. Sometimes, with chronic pain or emotional stress, we compartmentalize areas of our body as a coping mechanism. There are also microexpressions and areas of the face we might be completely unaware of—that we have learned to dissociate from. Over time we can lock away old feelings in the dungeons and subterranean aspects of our person.

In childhood we are often conditioned to disconnect from our gut feelings, heart feelings, and intuitions. Through the trials of our teenage years, it has become quite normalized to develop a subtle sense of shame in our bodies that can gradually cut off our ability to feel into them. And so, the process of coming into the ground of our body paradoxically can both create the most profound sense of safety and at the same time has the potential for awakening old patterns of emotion. In either case, the pathway of release is the same. It is a letting go—a release to the ground—a coming down to Earth and back to the present moment anew. Like Indra's Net of Jewels, all aspects of ourselves are reflected on our face. And so, Dien Chan can initiate entryway into all the layers of emotion we hold and grant release from these old patterns.

The initial Dien Chan exercises we've explored so far offer a simple way to make it easier to reconnect the head to the body and shift into this more grounded mode of being. The first step in working with trauma and in the re-patterning of any emotional issue begins with establishing this sense of calmness, groundedness, and safety. For this reason, it is not advised that you begin using Dien Chan in an emotionally aroused or upset state of mind. Rather, it's better to begin exploring these deeper techniques when we are in a relativity calm state, so we can first strengthen and fortify our groundedness and thereby avoid jumping headfirst into emotional volatility.

The physical space you're in can either aid or negate a feeling of safety, and so it's recommended to find a place where you won't be disturbed and feel naturally comfortable.

The concepts of titration and the window of tolerance are useful here, as they provide a practical principle for the healing process: the quickest path to healing is the slow path. Titration is related to alchemy. When we have a chemical substance that reacts in an explosive and volatile way, the quickest way to neutralize this substance is to slowly titrate the substance drop by drop. Each drop creates a fizz in our experience, but we gradually absorb and digest the substance with time. The volatile substance is a metaphor for volatile emotions, and the ground substance that dissolves emotion is a calm and equanimous state of mind.

If we were to try to dive headfirst into our deepest fear or anger it is highly likely that the experience will overwhelm us. It would be like combining the two alchemical substances all together at once—an explosion would occur. This metaphorical explosion usually presents in one of two ways: (1) being triggered, which is a common but not entirely helpful description of feeling activated and overwhelmed, and (2) dissociation, which is a checking out from one's felt experience and gives rise to myriad somatic sensations, most usually characterized by not feeling in one's body.

And so, the balancing act is to continuously gauge at what point we are liable to become overwhelmed. This tipping point is framed as our window of tolerance. Lasting healing occurs when we play within this somatic domain.

However, we shouldn't take these concepts too literally, as you will notice that sometimes our window of tolerance is much smaller than at other times, and sometimes the volatility of our emotions is also changeable. Again, by framing our emotions as substances we react to and are triggered by, or that are somehow fixed inside of us, we blind ourselves to the highly fluid and lightning-quick nature of consciousness.

This natural changeability is always occurring, even with old patterns. We never step in the same river twice, and so it is with emotion. They might seem and feel the same, but you are not the same person as you were when the emotional event was first initiated. There is what we remember about the original emotional event, and then there is what we re-create and layer upon it in each present moment. As Barrett says, "All memory is reassembly."

Therefore, our ability to remain mindful and pull ourselves back from the brink of being triggered or dissociated is the ongoing skill of what is often called emotional self-regulation. The continual coming back to the present moment can form a wedge of mindfulness that can help free us from the tendency to re-traumatize ourselves through remembrance.

It's an entirely natural experience to be overwhelmed with emotion, and sometimes it's entirely appropriate to be devastated by grief or blind with rage. But when these experiences become entrenched and we keep repeating them, or if they get submerged and locked away, this is when they can lead or contribute to the many chronic health disorders that besiege our society. And so, initially we need to just bring our bodies to rest, to give ourselves some grounding stability and safety. Then, when we are ready, we can bring some curiosity toward exploring where our boundaries lie, to how much we can fully embody and sit within the fullness of our lives.

The optimal grip is to embody both calmness and a sense of courage and curiosity. It's sometimes only by overstepping our window of tolerance that we discover where it actually is. The ability to draw ourselves back into our window of safety and calmness is a large part of the re-patterning of emotional habits. In this sense, our ability to move in and out of emotion with smoothness is a good marker of health. If we can feel angry and then easily come back to neutral, this quickly dissipates any emotional residue or charge, which would otherwise remain unintegrated in our felt body.*

When we apply self-massage techniques to our face, neck, and body there is a dynamic fundamentally different from receiving a massage from someone else. In the latter case we can release all control over our body, we can let go and be completely passive and limp. In self-massage we have a greater conscious participation in the felt sense of our body. For instance, it's very difficult to tickle yourself. This means we have greater control in how we explore and transform both the external stimulus to our body and the internal response.

Our consciousness plays a powerful role in self-massage, as the state of mind we bring to our touch can have a transformative effect on the holding patterns and emotional pathways of our body. Ironically, while

---

*This fluidity of felt emotion has an interesting correlate to what is termed *heart rate variability* (HRV). HRV is different from heart rate in that it doesn't measure the speed of the heartbeat, rather it measures the ability of the heart to change speed from one beat to the next. This in turn adapts and optimizes our heart function and blood circulation in response to our brain and body's continual energetic demands. When we look at a graph of HRV, we automatically assume that the steady, syncopated pattern is the sign of health and the erratic pattern is unhealthy. But actually, the more steady and rigid HRV becomes, the greater the risk of heart attack and stroke. Inversely, the more changeable the heart rate is in its second-to-second rhythm, the healthier we are. HRV is the easiest marker of vagal tone and has a striking parallel to the emotional flexibility that is characteristic of an optimal grip. In sum, be like water and you can flow and adapt to the tides of emotion that we are continuously buffered by. If we hold on too hard or can't let go of our emotions in real time, this rigidifies our experience of the world. Over time, this affects not only our physical health, but we come to see everything through the lens of our own anguish, resentment, or fear as well.

we must take control over the movement and pressure of our hands in self-massage, at the same to we are seeking to release control over the habitual expressions that keep our emotional patterns locked in the tissues of our face, head, or neck. It's like a playful dance between these different aspects of our person.

The key is to retain the feeling of calmness, safety, and equanimity while at the same time staying in touch with all the physical and emotional sensations that may be activated through our massage and presence within the body. This sounds more complicated than it is. It can be more simply described as using our body to support calmness in the mind and using calmness to explore and reassure the body.

This is also the secret to being able to fully receive massage from another—as pressure is applied, we are able to internally feel and release into the pressure, thereby participating with and assisting the masseur's intention, which is usually to increase circulation and release physical tension from our body. Inversely, if we tense our body when receiving massage, this increases the likelihood of pain, injury, or bruising.

While the physical act of touching our chin or forehead might elicit only the tiniest recognition of an emotional expression, it's actually these microexpressions that are linked to our bodies patterned responses. There is a subtlety involved in this process that takes a little time to feel in to. When we give our mind a more active role in self-care massage, this deepens the practice beyond establishing physical comfort and into inquiry and self-transformation. By continually increasing this questioning of our own faces we can shift our whole way of being toward renewal and re-imagination. We begin unmasking all the stories we tell ourselves about ourselves and start to awaken to a more truthful self-perception. This is akin to the old Zen task of searching for one's original face.

The first step to bringing our touch to the emotional layer of the face is to start bringing more awareness to the face-emotion connection while we practice self-massage. We don't just massage the face; we massage the mind through the face. By increasing our mindfulness, we can begin to feel not only the physical anatomy of the face but also the mental-emotional anatomy. Very often this reveals that we are holding on to so much tension in our face!

Even though the face has such a high density of nerve tissue, it's often the case that we're dissociated and disconnected from how our face actually feels. Usually it's only through touch that we realize how much tension we are holding. When people explore meditation, this is a common finding: that the face carries hidden tension, the release of which opens up more peaceful and spacious states of mind.

The previous four self-massage sequences can be revisited with this change of mind, and you will feel a subtle but noticeably different effect afterward. The deeper we engage the mind-body dynamic, the more important our intention becomes. Our intention should not simply be to clear away and release emotion but to remain present and equanimous in the face of emotional arousal. It's this presence of mind and the power of equanimity that unravels and dissolves emotional patterns. In practice, this translates to the quality of touch. When our touch is slow and light, it helps support a stronger mind-body connection.

Often, we can't feel the emotional tension in our face because we dislike our emotional patterns, and because of this aversion we often dissociate and become numb to what is there. If our touch is too quick and strong it can pass right through these layers of numbness. Rather than trying to force the tension out of our face, the more effective mind-set is to enfold our experience within a neutral awareness. If we can maintain equanimity or even generate kindness and self-compassion, we can gradually re-pattern our expressions. With time, our internal, emotional landscape will become more beautiful, and concordantly the complexion of our face will also grow into a more beautiful appearance.

The following sequences offer a deeper exploration into the emotional layers of our face. There are three basic techniques explored here:

holding, point pressing, and tapping. Each creates a slightly different feeling, but if we keep our intent and quality of awareness grounded and neutral, then each technique can create change in our emotional patterning.

✿ Light Touch for Connection and Sensitivity

The first sequence uses a very light touch to establish connection and build sensitivity to the entangled fabric of our faces. The tips of the first two fingers are very gently pressed into the skin, and then we release the pressure, so the fingers are just lightly resting with barely any pressure. This is the holding technique, and it heightens our ability to feel into the mind-body connection. The sequence is done as slowly as you like, but generally it's necessary to hold each point for at least five to ten seconds.

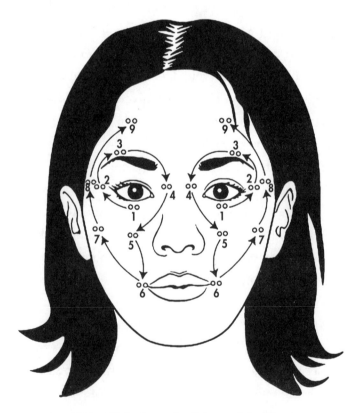

Figure 11.1. Areas for light-touch holding

1. Press, release, and hold the tips of the two fingers upon the ocular ridge just below the eyes.

2. Shift to the ocular ridge at the side of the eyes, just in front of the temples and at the edges of the eyebrow and eye.

3. Shift to hold the fingertips on the two points above the eye, on the upper edge of your eyebrows.

4. Hold the tip of the index finger in the point just inside and above the inner corner of the eye, holding the middle fingertips upon the crest of the nose.

5. Shift to hold the area just underneath the cheekbones and just outside the nostrils.

6. Shift to hold the points just under the outer corners of the lips. You can use three fingertips to cover the whole area of the chin.

7. Shift to hold the chewing muscles underneath the cheekbones and in front of the ears.

8. Shift to hold three fingertips upon the temples.

9. Shift to hold the area at the middle of the forehead above the eyes.

10. To finish, place one palm on the center of your chest and overlay the other palm, so you can feel the warmth of the hands on your chest and feel the breath and heartbeat within.

❀ Opening the Energy Gates of the Face

The second sequence introduces us to the stimulation and opening of the energetic points on the face. As has been discussed, within any square millimeter on the face lie potentially active points. You can tell if a point is active by noticing an increase of normal sensitivity—tenderness. This means the point will create a stronger effect through the brain, body, and mind. It can also be the case that points that are unusually insensitive or numb may be active or blocked, but this is less noticeable, so harder to feel. Places that lack feeling are often where we dissociate from emotion. Apart from these active points there are hundreds of Dien Chan points on the face that have specific actions and uses.

Unless otherwise stated, use the pad and fingertip of the index finger to press on these points. Press into the point slowly, gradually increasing the pressure over a count of three, so that after a few seconds you are pressing firmly and deeply on the point. As you do this, make a slow and long exhale. Your intention is clear and open, just being present with the feeling. Once all the breath is released, you can pause for a moment at the end of the exhale and then at the same speed slowly release the pressure as you take a slow breath in.

1. Slowly inhale and rest your fingertips upon the soft spaces just inside and above the inner corner of the eye (BL1/*Jing Ming*/Bright Eyes). The fingertips should feel as if they're pressing toward each other, squeezing the bridge of the nose.

2. Open the jaw wide and slowly press into the hollow space that opens just in front of the ear (SI19/*Ting Gong*/Listening Palace). Remember to go slowly and exhale fully. The fingertips should slowly dampen your sense of hearing.

3. Repeat step 1, pressing on BL1/*Jing Ming*/Bright Eyes as you exhale.

4. Open the first two fingers into a peace sign and place the tips of the middle fingers just outside the outer corner of the eye, in the space just on the edge of the ocular ridge (GB1/*Tong Zi Liao*/Bone of New Vision). Place the index finger directly behind this point, in the soft space just in front of the ear and above the jawbone (TB22/*He Liao*/ Singing Bone Harmony). Slowly press and release the middle fingers in concert with your breath and intention. Keep the fingers in place and slowly press the index fingers. Finally, come back with your third breath on the TB22/*He Liao*/Singing Bone Harmony point.

5. Place the right fingertip at the end of the crease of the right nostril (LI20/*Ying Xiang*/Welcoming Fragrance) and the left fingertip on the ocular ridge immediately below the center of the pupil (ST1/*Cheng Qi*/Receiving Tears). As you exhale, press the nostril firmly in, so that you can feel the edge of the nasal bone. Take a slow breath in as

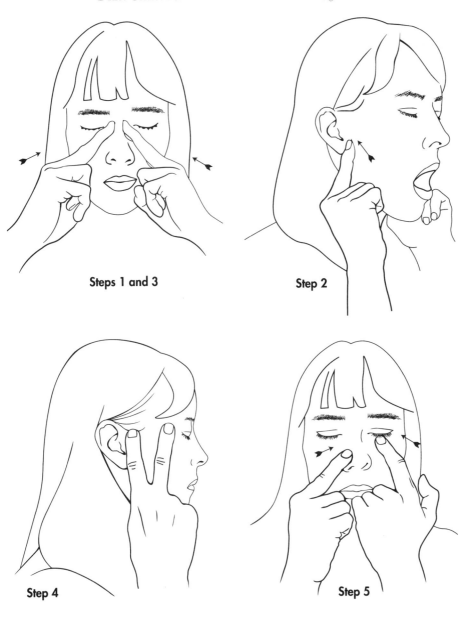

Figure 11.2. Opening the Energy Gates of the Face
Step 1, Pressing BL1/*Jing Ming*/Bright Eyes.
Step 2, Pressing SI19/*Ting Gong*/Listening Palace.
Step 4, Pressing TB22/*He Liao*/Singing Bone Harmony
alongside GB1/*Tong Zi Liao*/Bone of New Vision.
Step 5, Pressing LI20/*Ying Xiang*/Welcoming Fragrance
alongside ST1/*Cheng Qi*/Receiving Tears.

your release the nostril, and then press down on the ST1/*Cheng Qi*/ Receiving Tears point as you exhale.

6. Repeat step 5 on the other side.

7. Use the index finger middle knuckle of your dominant hand, pressing slowly but very firmly onto the point between the upper lip and the nose (Du26/*Ren Zhong*/Central Being). This should feel like you're pressing the lip into the point just above the two front teeth. Then use the same knuckle to press the point directly below on the crease of the chin (Ren24/*Cheng Jiang*/Broth of Life).

All the points you have opened are known as the entry-exit points, where the pathways of various channels meet and interlink. By stimulating and opening these points we disinhibit the blockages that tend to arise between the Wu Xing (Five Elements). These blockages can reflect the inability to shift from one emotion to the next or the resistance to shift out of an emotion.

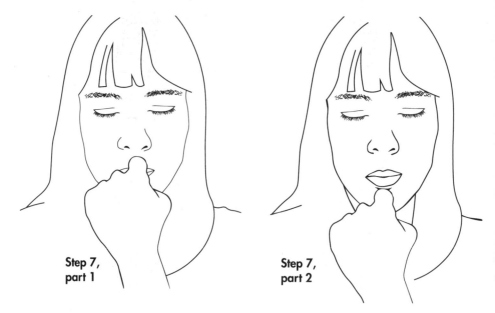

Step 7, part 1

Step 7, part 2

Figure 11.2. Opening the Energy Gates of the Face *(continued)*
Step 7, Pressing Ren24/*Cheng Jiang*/Broth of Life
and Du26/*Ren Zhong*/Central Being.

🪷 Tapping for Release and Transformation

The third sequence builds upon the last and can be used as an add-on or as a stand-alone practice. This sequence uses a different way of touching—gently tapping on each point in a fairly quick rhythm. The tip of the index or middle finger can be used, whichever feels more comfortable. The breath is natural, and more emphasis is placed on generating equanimity and calmness. The sequence starts with points at the top of the head and slowly works it ways down the face, the neck, and finally, the abdomen. With each point, keep tapping for a duration of five to twenty seconds, then move on. The tapping is light to medium in pressure, and the movement is best done either

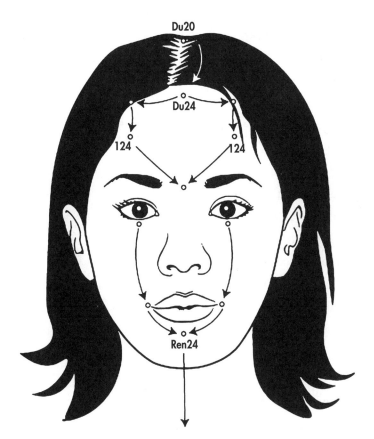

Figure 11.3. Tapping for emotional
release and transformation

from base of the knuckle or from the wrist, so that the elbow and shoulder are relatively still.

1. Begin tapping at the highest point on the crown of the head, between the tips of the ears (Du20). (See figure 11.3 on page 167 for an illustration of the following instructions.)
2. Shift to the point directly in front, just above the hairline (Du24). Then shift to tapping with both hands on the hairline points an inch lateral to Du24.
3. Shift downward to the two points in the middle of the forehead (point 124).
4. Shift to the third-eye point, using one finger.
5. Shift back to using two hands, gently tapping the points just below the center of the eye.
6. Slowly tap and move the fingertips downward toward the corners of the mouth.
7. Shift the tapping to the points just underneath the corners of the mouth, using both the index and middle fingers.
8. Shift to using one finger on Ren24/*Cheng Jiang*/Broth of Life, on the middle of the chin crease.
9. Shift directly down the centerline to the point at the base of the throat, then slowly tap down the centerline of the chest, either with all the fingertips of both hands or one fingertip.
10. Switch to using gently cupped palms, crossing the hands over and patting the opposite collarbones.
11. With one palm, pat down underneath the armpit and down toward the lower ribs. Follow with the other side.
12. Finish by gently patting down the abdomen and slowly come to a stop, holding the palms on the belly, and breathing slowly into it.

Although it may seem like there are too many points to remember, don't be overwhelmed—once you see the general pattern, it's quite simply moving from top to bottom, tracing the downward flow. Don't be overly concerned with being precisely on the correct point; rather the emphasis should be made, to maintain the felt connection through the body. Tapping the body and bringing a neutral awareness to each point can shift old patterns within our face and body. Finally, these points are not arbitrary, but at the same time they can be adjusted and changed according to your felt experience and intuition. For instance, you may wish to omit certain points at certain times—quickly brush over them—or spend a longer time with other points.

In the previous chapter I've highlighted equanimity as of primary importance in emotional well-being and in discovering the optimal grip of wei wu wei. Calmness opens us to curiosity, which in turn opens our eyes and senses to new possibilities. And so, calmness and equanimity are the prerequisites for emotional healing, for re-patterning our stories, and for harnessing the power of neuroplasticity.

However, there is a caveat in that each person has different degrees of access to their equanimity. It comes easier for some than others. Thankfully, equanimity is a quality of mind that can be cultivated, built up, and practiced in the same way that we can strengthen our vagal tone. Equanimity can be thought of not just as an emotion but as a biological strength that arises from a healthy heart. The physical parallel of equanimity is in our ability to physically relax and release into the pressure of touch.

The organ of the heart not only reflects the interoceptive feelings of how much physical pressure our body is under, but it also reflects our capacity for wisdom; that is, the embodied insight that emerges when we fully acknowledge the transience and impermanence of things. The clear light of emptiness is perceived through the heart. This inherent luminosity, the heart sense, heart intelligence, or the heart of the Dao, can enlighten us to the nature of emotional suffering. It can shift us from being embroiled in the tragedy of life to a kind of post-tragic presence that can withstand emotional turmoil. We all have different degrees of access to this kind of heart intelligence. In accordance with this, we also have different capacities for equanimity and resilience.

However, there is another way of working with emotion that can also re-pattern our old habits, albeit from a slightly different angle. This technique can be kept in mind for the self-massage practices given in this chapter, if you feel you need something more tangible to lean on in the face of emotional arousal. In a nutshell, while practicing Dien Chan, we can transform negative emotional arousal by self-generating positive mind-body states.

In the next chapter we'll look at how to generate these states and their role in healing. As we'll see, this is a practice that not only features in Eastern spiritual systems but is also apparent the world over, suggesting that it is an innate process we all naturally possess. Indeed, the ability to brighten a room and lift another's spirits is a normal part of most peoples' social lives. But this social instinct also plays an important role in personal healing and growth.

TWELVE

The Two Faces of Buddha

The face is a hologram, not just of the body and its internal structure and function, but it is really a holographic interpretation of your soul and your soul's growth.

LILLIAN BRIDGES

When our hearts are small, our understanding and compassion are limited, and we suffer. We can't accept or tolerate others and their shortcomings, and we demand that they change. But when our hearts expand, these same things don't make us suffer anymore. We have a lot of understanding and compassion and can embrace others. We accept others as they are, and then they have a chance to transform.

THICH NHAT HANH

When all the points and areas of tension are released from the face, a cascade effect down through the body is created. This downward flow is a motion of reconnection, a grounding and increased awareness of our felt body. We can feel the nuanced microrhythms of our heart with more clarity; we can feel the breath as more expansive and open; we can feel in to the depths of our body with more assuredness.

This pathway from our face to our heart to our belly mirrors the course of the vagus nerve, and as such could be thought of as the pathway of release from all stress and anxiety. It's for this reason the vagus is sometimes called the antianxiety nerve. The stronger our vagal tone, the stronger our ability to remain calm and lucid. Vagal tone stops us from feeling overwhelmed by the surging of emotion. However, this is not the full picture. In the same way that consciousness and personhood can't be reduced to the physical structure of the brain; calmness and resilience are more than simply having strong vagal tone. For this reason, it's helpful to explore other ways of looking at the embodiment of emotion.

In Chinese medicine, the most detrimental and destructive of emotions are often thought to be anger, rage, irritation, and the plethora of feelings that are related. The direction of anger is taken to be like fire, an upward blazing, scorching the heart and boiling the head. This upward surging into the head is counteracted by what I have called the downward flow of the vagus nerve. In qigong practice, this motion is called sinking the qi and is a primary skill, for it draws us down from our heads and develops our connection to the Earth.

However, this downward flow is also a natural and fundamental part of becoming an adult, and through our social learning as a child, we naturally hone this skill of not flying into a tantrum whenever we are displeased. It reflects the development of both our emotional regulation and our interoception. This is why we naturally say cool *down,* settle *down,* and slow *down,* because this is the direction that counteracts the emotions that most viscerally unbalance us. Such is life that we must keep relearning the basics, or as one of my teachers describes it, "advanced techniques are basic techniques mastered."

Coming to rest in the center of our body is synonymous with the cultivation of a calm presence. The feeling of calmness has a spectrum to it, and at the deep end of this spectrum is this quality of equanimity, of being able to remain calm amid the storm. It's this level of calmness that can re-pattern and heal old dynamics of emotional stress and trauma. A full-bodied deep sense of calmness can gradually re-pattern our nervous system toward feeling safe, even amid discomfort. The deepening of feeling safe in our body gradually loosens the hold of stress. When we have strong equanimity, our minds and nervous systems are protected from the re-traumatization that can occur when releasing old emotional patterns.

So much of chronic pain, anxiety, and trauma arises from the nervous system being on hyperalert, of feeling constantly under threat. It's often the case that stress and anxiety are similar to anger in that they have this upward direction into the head. When we are in fight-or-flight mode, our eyes and ears open to full alert, our face contracts, and we are less tuned to the digestive and integrative energies of the body. In fact, our digestive system switches off when our body is in full-on survival mode, which explains the common stress connection to IBS (irritable bowel syndrome), digestive issues, and sexual and gynecological issues. The vagus nerve is known as the antianxiety nerve not only because it also counteracts the misperceptions of danger, but because it reconnects us to our felt sense of the body and switches on the healing and regenerative capacity of our body.

Interestingly, this sense of feeling connected to our body opens up a feeling of being connected to the world around us. When we are calm and embodied, it is much easier to connect with other people. It's as if our minds are not contracted inward but extended outward. And because we feel safe and embodied, this extension of our awareness is not scanning for threats but is sensitized to the musicality and creativity around us. We are more open to the spontaneous inter-being of others. This connection doesn't stop at the social level, though, but extends into everything our perception touches: we shift toward a world of inter-being and resonance and away from a world of fragmented and disconnected things.

The psychiatrist and philosopher Iain McGilchrist has made groundbreaking work in showing how these two different ways of seeing the world, as holistic or as fragmented, are both fundamental to human nature and also descriptive of the way each hemisphere of the brain sees the world. The left brain dissects the world into parts; the right brain connects the world into wholes. Although the reductionist and analytic way of thinking has incredible uses, it's the right brain that holds the key, for it can bring everything back together again into a coherent picture. It's the right brain that can grasp the big picture and contend with complexity.

Interestingly, it's also the right side of the brain that is in stronger resonance with the vagus nerve, thus enabling both a sense of feeling wholly embodied and a perception of inter-being and embeddedment. What this means is that the downward flow of connecting to our body not only soothes our nervous system and cultivates a sense of calmness, but it also reorients our brain and perception toward wholeness. In other words, embodiment doesn't isolate us from everything outside our skins but instead opens and connects us to the wholeness in nature. This has profound implications for our emotional lives. As the storyteller Martin Shaw tells it: "Relatedness breeds love, and love can excavate conscience. Conscience changes the way we behave."[1]

A profound and creative reorientation is brought to our lives when we can relate toward the world as a place of familiarity and kinship, as if the whole planet is a shared home to all its inhabitants. We look upon ourselves and others with eyes of friendship and kindness rather than suspicion and alienation. This can defuse the emotional knots of anger, irritation, resentment, and all the emotions that seem to divide us.

Our right-brain hemisphere has the capacity to bring things into relatedness, to make things whole again. This is a big deal, because it's not always easy to access the depths of calmness and equanimity that can shift old emotional patterns. When we are caught up in the storm of emotional arousal and feelings of overwhelm, it may be too challenging to maintain our equanimity. In such times we can find support in the power of love. Our capacity to generate states of love can de-tribalize our minds and open us to emotional healing and to a process of peacemaking within and without. Love can elevate us toward wisdom and away from the very human tendency to scapegoat, ostracize, and frame fellow humans as *other*.

The ability to draw connection and build relatedness is universal in humans; it's a core part of our nature. I would suggest that this innate tendency toward forming relationship is not only human but is extended throughout nature as well. Taken further, I suggest we expand and reframe our idea of love as both human and more-than-human, as fundamental to all life on Earth.

Although, at first our connection with love for our own body or with the world around us might seem precarious or even lacking, we can take comfort in the message of reassurance that the world's wisdom traditions convey: the inherent nature of the world is of total acceptance and love. No matter who or where we are, we are always continuously embedded in this natural reverberation of acceptance and love.

This might seem far-fetched to those who only see the brutality and terror in the world or see nature purely as a place of cold alienation and hostility. This idea can seem like a radical affront to that part of us that has been wounded by the world. But consider the people who have delved most deeply into the nature of the mind: the seers, sages, and wisdom keepers; they refute this simplistic picture of life as only terror and misery. It should also be noted that often these people have endured great suffering and know the pain of the world very well.

They use words like *unconditional forgiveness, boundless compassion,* and *all-embracing bliss.* These are examples of what the Irish mystic

John Moriarty calls the "betrayals of language," for they are extremely limited descriptions of some of the experiences that can emerge when we overstep the boundaries between self and world and come into greater relatedness. The face is one such boundary. It's both a symbol of who we are and acts as a stage of transparency for the nature of the world. This is the implication of finding your original face. It's the discovery of the face's mythical dimension, that which unites the personal to the universal.

This is one of the reasons why the human face holds such significance within religious and spiritual motifs, for it reflects both that which separates us and that which unites us. The face conveys and transmits both our personal love and Love at its grandest and most mysterious.

Releasing contraction from our face helps us return and reconnect to our body. This letting go of tension from the face is one pathway into the downward flow, into a state of calmness and equanimity.

However, there is another pathway into the downward flow that we can access when calmness and equanimity are elusive. Instead of letting go, we can emphasize a giving in toward kindness, love, and goodwill. Specifically, this giving in is a softening and release from the chest and heart, a physical and mental act of surrender that can bring us home to the body when our masks are too tightly clenched. It can melt the tension from the face in an indirect way, opening a slightly different dimension to the downward flow.

This dimension is based not on equanimity but on love. If we frame the simple act of listening, of being present with ourselves, as a form of kindness, it's a small step to notice how this act can generate a feeling of love. Gently placing our attention and giving in to the space around our heart can especially spark this self-generation of love. Sometimes this is called the inner smile or the practice of loving-kindness.

These two movements, the letting go of the face and the giving in of the heart, are two different pathways into relaxation. We are either releasing and letting go from the surface of the face down into the body or surrendering from the heart and allowing this softening to melt away tension from the face. It's either a top-down relaxation or a bottom-up relaxation. Although subtle, this gives us some options for exploring how to reconnect to our bodies.

Just like a fractal pattern that is reflective of a much larger movement in the world, this interplay of love and equanimity is both an inherent feature of our personal biology and is at play in much larger spheres around us. Again, there is a betrayal of language here, as what we are really referring to is not the normal conception of love or calmness but instead a much grander process more akin to gravity or light.

The two sides of the face have a unique resonance with these grander notions of love and equanimity. Iain McGilchrist has explored how the two hemispheres of the brain parallel the two sides of the face. The right side of the face is controlled by the left brain, while the left side of the face is controlled by the right brain. He suspects this was intuitively apprehended in the ancient iconography of Buddhism.[2]

This was first documented in the 1930s by William Empsom, who spent many years visiting and studying Buddhist sculptures and temples throughout the Far East.[3] Empsom noticed that in a great many depictions of the Buddha's face there was a noticeable variance between the left and right side of the face. This asymmetry is curious, and his initial thought was that if the Buddha's face was depicted only in the blissful detachment of deep samadhi—the totally equanimous enlightened state—then worshippers might feel a little disconnected and alienated from the Buddha. And so, he suggested that one side of the face was depicted to give an expression of love and compassion, to conjure a bond and aspiration in devotees.

Although this suggests that early Buddhists might be partaking in some kind of idolatry, it may be that there was a more complex intuition behind this asymmetry, one that McGilchrist suggests could point back toward the nature of the brain and mind.

My own understanding of what Buddhists call unconditional love and equanimity suggests these are not simply emotions in the everyday sense. Instead, these feelings are more fundamental to both human nature and the nature of mind-at-large. Indeed, this is how Buddhists describe these emotions, as the four Brahmavihara: the sublime abidings of love, equanimity, compassion, and appreciative joy. These are framed as higher orders of emotion. They're states that humans can participate in but at the same time are also fundamental to the nature of reality. We can abide within them, as if they are already here.

If we look further into these states, we can see that love, compassion, and appreciative joy are somewhat related. Indeed, compassion naturally arises when a loving mind touches the suffering of another, and joy arises when a loving mind touches the happiness of another. But equanimity is unique among the four Brahmavihara. My meditation teacher describes equanimity as the highest of the stars, that from which true love and compassion emerge. Equanimity is the closest mental state we have to the pristine nature of emptiness. It can therefore be thought of as a way to come into resonance with Shen Ming—the natural blueprint for our growth and healing.

I suspect that this primordial interplay between love and equanimity can be seen on the two sides of the Buddha's face, and also between the right- and left-brain hemispheres.

In both Dien Chan and Chinese medicine there is a yin-yang relationship between the two sides of the body. However, this is one of the main points of contrast between the two traditions, for in Chinese medicine, the right side of the body is yin and the left yang—whereas in Dien Chan, the right side of the face is yang and left yin. This is a slightly minor point, as yin and yang are never absolute, always relative, reversing, and transforming. Therefore, if you overlay the yin-yang symbol onto the face you will notice that black and white appear on both sides. Likewise, each side of the body can be further divided into yin and yang, and so there is always a relative nature when we speak of these concepts—never absolute.

In practice, one of the principles of Dien Chan is that the points are always stimulated on the left side first, followed by the right side. In point selection, there is always a movement from left to right. To me, this suggests we're highlighting the right side of the brain, which is holistic and integrative, and carrying over these qualities into the more fragmented and particular nature of our selves.

If we look at Vietnamese acupuncture, the first point that is needled is considered the master point, and the second and third points are considered emissary points. So, in Dien Chan we're highlighting the soothing intelligence of the right hemisphere and carrying it toward the analytic vexations of the left hemisphere. This brings a sense of balance to both sides of the body. Because the right hemisphere strongly connects to the vagus nerve and interoception, this also brings us into a more holistic sense of embodiment, connecting and balancing both the vertical and horizontal planes of our mind-body.

This is an important takeaway—our sense of physical and mental-emotional balance comes from a synchrony between both the left and right sides of the body, brain, and also along the vertical access between the face, heart and belly. The Dien Chan techniques we've explored so far help us find this balance; they allow us to return to our center. Furthermore, I would add that our capacity for calmness and love play an equal part in our embodiment. This is because these feelings are not just human feelings but percolate through and connect us to the greater relatedness of the world. Love and calmness describe the natural resting state of humans and are also present within nature-at-large. When we find our centerline—our Zhong Qi—we are connected to nature's regenerative and healing impulse. Therefore, learning how to generate and strengthen our capacity for calmness, equanimity, and love is integral to our health.

Connecting into an unconditional form of love may seem as challenging as being able to drop into an unshakable state of equanimity. However, it's not necessary to be a perfectionist with these states—all that is needed is a hint of a smile and the gentlest inclination of the heart to set in motion a positive chain reaction through our nervous system, mind, and perception.

This chain reaction resonates beyond the body, too. This small prompt can be made entirely with our imagination, it can be made with the slightest of smiles, or with a slow, long sigh of an out-breath. In qigong, this is known as hollowing the chest or emptying the heart and is both a physical relaxation of this area of the body and a concurrent relaxation of the mind. Dien Chan self-care massage can help release these areas under the chin, through the neck and chest. If we bring a positive attitude to our touch, this will create a more powerful effect, especially when the intention is toward emotional balance.

If we want to bring in a more substantial form of self-generation, we can use intentional speech, which is known variously as affirmation, invocation, mantra, and prayer. The resonance of the voice helps open the throat and reconnect the head and heart. This is how the Buddhist practice of loving-kindness is more formally taught, through mantra and intentional speech.

Saying the words, with both our internal and external voice, "May I be happy and peaceful," offers a prompt toward self-love, toward surrendering into this feeling in this moment. Keeping the intention sustained with embodied mindfulness can gradually increase this feeling until it's as if it's permeating the whole mind-body. At first, the intention and feeling are as broad as possible, as if we are entering a realm of love rather than just thinking something up. This is important, as for most people there are many aspects of their body and personhood they don't fully love or accept. But it's entirely possible to generate a feeling of love toward oneself, even if there are contradictory feelings at play, like we're offering a hand of friendship to all the forlorn parts of ourselves. A helpful stepping-stone toward a greater embrace of this feeling is the ongoing process of forgiveness. As forgiveness unfolds, relatedness is reestablished, and the feeling of loving-kindness starts to come unstrained. Eventually, love becomes completely effortless, a state we can naturally abide within.

This brings us to an adjoining practice that can also be extremely helpful for our purposes. Known by the wonderful name of Hoʻoponopono, this practice has traditionally been used for social healing in Hawaii.[4] A simplified version of the practice involves the invocation of four statements:

> *I'm sorry.*
> *Please forgive me.*
> *Thank you.*
> *I love you.*

The intention for these words is directed initially inward, saying: *I'm sorry* to myself, *please forgive me* to myself, *thank you* to myself, *I love you* to myself. When repeated and with sustained intention, this simple sequence can help turn around and transform negative spirals of emotion. It also has an uncanny ability to affect not only our own relationships but those of other people, too.

Both loving-kindness and Hoʻoponopono are powerful tools for shifting our relationship with our mind-body. Although they might seem very simple, don't underestimate the potency of self-forgiveness, love, and gratitude. They're revolutionary for the heart. There are studies that show that a loving-kindness or gratitude practice can have a powerful effect on both the vagus nerve and on neuroplasticity.

In 2013, research was done to study how loving-kindness meditation affected vagal tone, and how it promoted positive emotions and improved physical health. The study found that sending loving-kindness toward oneself and toward others whether loved one, friend, or enemy, is the key to improved vagal tone.[5]

These emotions can change who we are at a fundamental level. By learning to generate a sense of strong loving-kindness toward ourselves, we can affect our physical health in profound ways. It's a deceptively powerful practice. Dien Chan can help unblock the connections between the face and heart, which in turn can open us toward a greater and greater sense of embodiment, centeredness, and love.

It is often said that you can only truly love another when you have learned to love yourself. And we can only truly love ourselves when we can forgive ourselves. If we harbor any self-loathing or shame, this mutes the full intensity of true love, by which I mean complete acceptance and unconditional love. This doesn't mean we can't develop kindness and positive self-regard, but we are limiting ourselves from the full healing effect that is inside of us. This is why forgiveness plays such an important part of both Metta and Ho'oponopono.

Forgiveness starts with admitting we have made mistakes, both knowingly and unknowingly—that we are not perfect. Crucially, all of our past mistakes, which stop us from feeling unconditional love, are not the result of us being bad people. Our mistaken ways of acting, speaking, and thinking are not the result of any innate personal deficiency. This would be framing ourselves as a fixed individual rather than as a person who is interconnected and interdependent with our social circle and environment, which is always changing and capable of growth. Instead, all our mistakes simply come from confusion.

Confusion, ignorance, and inattentiveness are the reality of what we call evil. Understanding this shadow aspect of ourselves can gift us insight into the seemingly evil behavior of others. Behind all such behavior we'll find troubled and traumatized souls. This way of seeing deeply into the cause of things is essential for comprehending the greater interconnectivity of trauma in our societies.

When we admit that we have some personal confusion when it comes to life and the various predicaments in which we find ourselves, that we haven't got it all figured out, then suddenly the mistakes and misjudgments we've made in the past become less heartbreaking. And when we realize that everybody else is also quite confused, then we see that the responsibility for hurtful behavior isn't as simple as one bad person but that we as people are intertwined through the actions and words of others.

Therefore, restraining from blaming other people and ourselves unties the heavy bonds of suffering that keep cycling through our families and communities.

This simple intention—*Do not blame others*—is the defining principle of an infamous movement of emotional healing that exploded through northern China in the late nineteenth and early twentieth centuries. Known as the Shan Ren Dao system, it was spearheaded by Wang Fengyi (1864–1937), a remarkable neo-Confucian educator and healer. Although from a Mongol peasant background in the harsh environment of the Far North, throughout his life he gathered a large following due both to his ethical integrity (for instance, his work helped establish more than seven hundred schools for girls) and for the many people he helped heal from sickness and disease.

At the heart of his message was that "all healing comes from the heart," that emotions are the primary cause of disease. His healing work didn't use any medicine or acupuncture but instead brought people and families together and used ritual storytelling, discussion, and what might be called group therapy to turn the hearts of sick people. He's renowned for helping people heal severe physical illness by catalyzing and releasing emotions.

While the Shan Ren Dao system is certainly embedded within that particular social time and environment, its principles and ethos bear relevance for us all. Learning to let go of the ill will we have for other people and ourselves can have a profound effect on our health and lives. A big part of this process hinges on forgiveness and acceptance.

The unwillingness to forgive and accept is often reflected by a hardening of our faces. The emotional dynamic between the face and the heart, between each side of the face, and between our own face and that of others, can be harnessed to soften and release the old patterns we carry. In this sense, Dien Chan can be of assistance with the inner work of emotional alchemy we engage in.

A special mention should be made of the pitfalls and misinterpretations that words like self-love and forgiveness can sometimes arouse. It can't be denied that modern culture is fine-tuning the art of narcissism to ever new heights. When we speak of generating self-love, it's helpful to distinguish between healthy, positive self-regard and narcissism. The sense of pride we have for ourselves, or any type of superiority that we might give ourselves, is a good indicator that our self-love might be slightly enmeshed with other emotions. The more we feel unconditional love, the less *self* stands in the way.

Likewise, when we forgive ourselves for our mistakes without actually realizing they were indeed mistakes, we risk a continuation of harmful behavior. This also applies to forgiving other people—it's premature to forgive the abuser while the abuse is happening . . . we must extract ourselves from harmful and life-threatening situations. The Christian rhetoric of turning the other cheek, while noble in principle, has also enabled much emotional abuse and suffering.

Both self-love and forgiveness are supported by clearly seeing into our deeper nature, our confusion and ignorance, and holding a clear resolve from falling back into harmful behavior and ways of thinking. The generation of these positive feelings, within our hearts and minds, helps us refrain from thinking badly about other people or harboring future resentment.

The pitfall of not clearly seeing into our shadow side is that practices such as loving-kindness or Ho'oponopono can become a form of spiritual bypassing, of dissociating from the discomfort of our own wrongdoing, confusion, and ignorance. This subtle distinction means we can truly untangle the emotional charge we carry rather than simply elevating ourselves above such feelings.

It should be emphasized that all these practices play out as an ongoing process and that a large part of the process is cutting ourselves some slack, realizing we are all works in process and all have our blind spots. Softening and accepting the emotions as they are clears space for strengthening our capacity to act with kindness and love for others.

Both the loving-kindness and Ho'oponopono practices start with our self-relationship before extending outward to others. Once we have established a stronger connection with our bodies and personhood, we may notice that the world around us is more vividly felt, that we can face the world not in an oppositional or predatory way but in a collaborative and co-creative way.

The changes in how we position our boundaries between self and world is a key aspect of trauma and also of embodiment more generally. One of the defining symptoms of trauma and PTSD is dissociation, but this same symptom is incredibly common to a lesser degree in a vast number of the population. It is like an unknown unknown—we usually don't feel when we disconnect from our bodies because there is no feeling. And it's only when we learn to come back in touch with all the locked-away parts of our physicality that we notice how much we've missed. Often it is only when we touch the body that we notice how much tension we carry. Human touch has an important role to play in reestablishing healthy boundaries. In the next chapter we will explore this common experience of boundary dissolution from some unusual angles.

THIRTEEN

· ·

Embodiment &
Disembodiment

*When the shoe fits, the foot is forgotten, when the belt fits,
the belly is forgotten.*

CHUANG TZU

Every day without fail a very strange thing happens to all of us. When
the sun sets and darkness engulfs us, we lie down, close our eyes, and
leave our body behind. This everyday occurrence is so normalized that
we rarely stop and question the strangeness of sleeping and dreaming. We can explain to ourselves that our biology necessitates sleep to
recover our energy and heal our body. But the actual experience of sleep
remains one of life's strangest things. For we not only completely dissociate from our body, but we also enter a dreamtime landscape where
time and space are completely different from waking life and our imagination presides. Even stranger than this is the fact that we are so habituated to this process that it barely warrants any attention.

The way we become normalized to weird things is both a functional
aspect of our brain and a key process that can be reversed to transform
patterns of stress and emotion. Strictly speaking, everything in life is

extremely weird. It only becomes normal because of repetition, and this normalizing effect means that as we pay less attention to our everyday reality, it becomes the background norm and allows us to focus in on what we need without distraction. All that's in the background periphery of our senses is literally a prediction that our brain is constructing for us so we can harness and direct our brain power toward what needs the most attention. As the weird becomes normalized, we in turn feel less challenged by the unknown aspects of life and form a bubble of safety to live within. This necessary management of our energy and our perplexity enables us to function well but can also restrict our sense of wonder and awe, in effect hindering our ability to explore what's outside of our knowledge.

Novelty is presented to us by all the unknown happenings of the world, and this triggers the brain's power of neuroplasticity, which is the brain's ability to rewire itself and update our experience and model of reality. Neuroplasticity is also generated through mindfulness and the simple act of paying close attention—for if we pay close attention to what is normal, we can learn to see through the ordinary into the extraordinary.[1] This is described by the philosopher Arthur Danto as "the transfiguration of the commonplace." It is well summed up by Heraclitus's adage of "never stepping in the same river twice."

Hence, our ability to be curious is the prerequisite for states of awe, wonder, and inspiration. These states of being play a vital role in personal growth and healing. Therefore, in the first decade of life our brains are exploding in plasticity, and as babies and children we are continuously blown away and enthralled by the world.

Once we can effectively model our reality, we no longer need to spend so much energy trying to apprehend our immediate situation as our brain starts to rely on its own predictions and models of the world. If we were to stop every time we're struck by the weirdness of life, we would never leave a baby's state of enthrallment. By learning to home in on what's most relevant to us, we can streamline our ability to act effectively in the world. This means we ignore all the sights and sounds that are normalized for us; they become a hazy background as we focus in on our personal priorities, which helps our brain process the vast amount of information that is constantly bombarding us.

Unfortunately, as the cognitive scientist Donald Hoffman succinctly points out, "our perceptions and models of reality are built primarily for survival rather than truth."[2] We don't see the world as it really is, but we perceive and make sense of the world according to what is relevant for our life. Our sensemaking apparatus is wonderfully adaptable, and we must indeed continually adapt to the world to survive, but this gift of adaptability also makes us incredibly prone to self-deception. We can easily become engrained in patterns of thinking and moving that aren't simply false but are detrimental to our health and growth. A lack of inspiration and wonder degrades both our quality of life and physical health. This is why Einstein famously stated that "imagination is more important than knowledge. Knowledge is limited. Imagination encircles the world."

It's not just our experience of the external world that's largely a product of our brain's predictive modeling; our experience of our body falls in and out of focus, too. The theologian Ivan Illich describes this relationship to our body as shifting between the *anatomical* body and the *felt* body.[3] As the name suggests, when we relate to the body through an anatomical lens, we are not engaging with our lived experience; we are not actually feeling our heart as it is at this moment. Instead, it's more like we are thinking about our body, and our thinking relies heavily on the predictive habits of our brain. This saves our brain some energy, but the downside is that we are cut off from being fully in touch with our body.

This subtle distinction between *thinking about* and *feeling within* is actually very important for healing. When we attend to our body with the full focus of our interoceptive sensitivity, we can powerfully activate the body's innate healing power. Interoception allows us to feel the background tone of our body, and this is where the patterns of stress, emotion, and trauma reside. It's important to know that interoception is a live process; it's always changing and never set in stone, like an anatomy textbook. Our organs are continuously changing their shape! The cellular makeup of the body is continually renewing.

Because of this continual renewal, the felt body can never be fully known because it remains open to the unknown becoming's of the present moment. We're not so much static human beings as we are human happenings, perpetually open to change and renewal. And because life is so wondrously complex, we have to switch off from this reality to maintain a sense of normalcy. Being open to the unknown engages a certain faculty of the imagination, and this can be a catalyst for both anxiety and delight. It's also closely linked to our bodies' natural impulse for healing and regeneration.

Being fully open to our bodies takes both curiosity and some boldness. To look upon ourselves as an unknown takes both imagination and courage. To become a question unto ourselves is indeed asking, "What is my original face?"

It can feel a bit risky to admit that we don't know and relinquish the part of us that is comfortable in its certainty. To dwell in the uncertainty of the felt body is to momentarily surrender the anatomical and analytical way of being. This is a completely different game to that of reasoning and acquiring knowledge. Our felt body, like our experience of the present moment, can never be fully known; it can only be felt. And if we honestly and openly engage our felt body, we can feel ourselves as ever new. The way in which we participate with this ever-new aspect of ourselves can change our experience of embodiment. It can re-pattern the old habits of our physical and emotional posture.

By paying attention to our body, we can actively change our health. Interoception strengthens vagal tone. And when we shift away from the normalized and slightly bored sense of our bodies, our curiosity can change our experience from a collection of separate bodily parts to feeling ourselves as a pulsing, breathing whole. This change in attention has tangible consequences for our health and embodiment. Our body can change from feeling dull and heavy to light and spacious.

If you bring your awareness to the felt experience of our heart—the inexplicable rhythm in our chest—we can notice the heart not only as a chunk of anatomy but as vividly connected to our whole body as well. We can feel the whole body through the heart in the same way that when we touch any part of the body we are also touching the whole. By sparking this kind of curiosity into our body we're seeding positive change for our health.

As has been mentioned, the felt body, which is accessed through interoception, is intimately involved in emotional well-being and vagal tone. Specifically, when we place a gentle awareness on the heart, we can generate a type of brain-heart coherence that benefits both heart function and whole-body health.* But that's not all; feeling our body as a whole can change our perception, bringing us in touch with the wholeness in nature.

This spectrum of embodiment between what is known and abstract and what is felt and immanent is a continual dance and balance. Both culturally and individually, we all have our habits of embodiment, posture, and thinking. By learning to change our physical posture, facial expression, and the way we move and gesture, we'll notice that our thinking, mood, emotion, and perception of the world also change.

If you close your eyes and quiet your senses from the world, and then focus all your attention on a thought so completely that you become absorbed in it, you might notice that both the physical world and your physical body can seem to disappear. This happens all the time when people stare at computers. The old Daoist trickster Chuang Tzu

---

*For more information on heart-brain coherence, see the pioneering work of the Heart Math Institute.

noted this tendency to forget our body when there is nothing imping-
ing on it. It's only after we have suffered a period of illness that we
notice how good it feels to simply be alive and healthy. Again, if we
were to be constantly amazed by the weirdly beautiful structure of
our hands or the deliciousness of wiggling our feet, we would never
get anything done! And so, we become normalized to having a body
and a fixed sense of self, when a more truthful reality shows that our
body and sense of self are in continual flux. This reflects something
fundamental to our existence—the balance we must make between
maintaining a safe normality and being open to novelty, risk, wonder,
and uncertainty.

Our experience of inhabiting a body can be quite different from person to person. When someone lives an intellectual life or is constantly
absorbed in daydreaming or abstraction, we say they live in their heads.
This ability to become lost in abstract thought and cognition not only
changes our relationship with our bodies into a top-down dynamic, but
it also means we can lose touch with the body altogether. We become
numb to the nuances and tastes of our internal space. This is actually
a mode of embodiment that Western culture has shifted toward more
and more over the past millennia. The lifework of historian F. Edward
Cranz makes a strong case that there was a type of interiorization of the
mind that made significant headway during the eleventh and twelfth
centuries. His thesis, which he called the reorientation of the Western
mind, is that people in Europe at this time began to separate their
abstract internal experience from the sense of being embedded within
the world.[4] At the crux of this reorientation was the way we communicate and make sense of the world—our language.

The work of Ivan Illich supports and convincingly details some of
the possible causes for this, tracing it back to the creation of universities and the division of medicine from philosophy during the eleventh
through the twelfth centuries. He says that "through the separation of
medicine and philosophy the interpretation of the felt body was replaced

by the external observation and manipulation of the anatomised body. Philosophy was deprived of the body, and the body was deprived of its cosmic belonging." He also describes how our cultural practice of literacy played an important role in this. Although being literate seems utterly normal to us now, it can't be understated how powerful this psychotechnology was in transforming our culture and self-understanding. Before the eleventh century, books were primarily read aloud; the texts, which were mostly religious, we're invoked by breathing life into them with our spoken voice.[5] As we began to read books purely in our heads, a more interiorized and abstract mode of being was created, one that created untold benefits but also pushed toward a severance between the mind and body and a somatic separation between self and the natural world.

Interestingly, this same period in Chinese history saw the most significant cultural change to literacy as well. Throughout the Song Dynasty, there was an explosion in growth, creating a massive revival of both industry, culture, philosophy, and medicine. Alongside the incredible wealth this brought, there was also a similar opening of universities in the form of the national examination system, which was open to all citizens. This opened education and literacy to a much broader audience, and, therefore, a similar claim could be made as to what happened in the West.[6] This movement into the head, and in our modern times into the brain, reflects a kind of cultural dissociation from being fully in touch with our bodies and with the full sensuality of the world.

It's only in the past few decades that the word *dissociation* has been used to describe this disconnecting from our felt sense of the body. Dissociation is usually framed as a pathological symptom of PTSD. However, this obscures the wider cultural context and also the wide variety of experiences that could be labeled as dissociation. What could be called mild dissociation or transient dissociation is incredibly common in all peoples, and this doesn't simply reflect the hidden epidemic of trauma in our society but also a more fundamental dynamic between mind and body.

The trauma specialist Ellert Nuijenhuis says, "The tendency to link dissociation only to negative symptoms is wrong. It's too limited and uninclusive."[7] This is because there are different forms of dissociation, some of which are indeed negatively connected to stress and trauma, and others that are not only positive but also integral to a full experience of life. Sleeping and dreaming are one example of this. A broad description of *dissociation* is "a disruption of our normal conscious state." It can also be descriptive of where we are placed on a spectrum of consciousness. At one end of the spectrum, we are fully embodied, heavy, and dense; at the other end of the spectrum, we are fully disembodied, light, and ethereal. Within this spectrum, we can experience many different modes of being. The ability to shift among these different modes of being is a skill that supports both survival, resilience, and what could be called the shamanic, creative, or visionary arts. Notice how there is a cultural presumption that a healthy person is individualized and has a clear and distinct boundary between what is *me* and what is *other*.

In the West, we have become so hyper-individualized that we have lost the wisdom of our relational nature. This doesn't mean that we have become non-relational but rather that we have collectively come to regard competition and rivalry as inherently superior to collaboration and dialogue. Our relationship with nature is a monologue, and our self-inquiry assumes we are solitary units of consciousness. Of course, the idea of appropriate boundaries and having self-sovereignty is an important part of growing into an adult, but on a broader scale a more truthful reality shows that our bodies are extremely porous to both our physical and social environments. A true self-sovereignty is humbled by and in service to the greater kingdoms that encompass us. If we're not humbled by anything, then we become like a tyrant to ourselves and others.[8]

Therefore, rather than assuming a fixed boundary between self and other, a healthier and more helpful sense of sovereignty lies in being able to appropriately adapt our boundaries to our changing situation. The discovery of the microbiome and the virome in the past few decades has been revolutionary—it shows that on a fundamental basis there is no strict dividing line between what is me and what is other. Every molecule of fragrance that enters our breath for a brief moment connects and binds to our brain; we unite with everything we breathe. A similar thing happens with everything we absorb into our mind-body. Because of this, our health is interdependent with our environment and community. This realization of being constituted by other things and other people occurs to many in their midlife when they realize they've perfectly replicated the mannerisms and foibles of their parents.

To effectively hold our individual sovereignty in balance with our relational nature requires the wisdom of being able to hold multiple orders of truth all at once. This is most readily achieved by remaining open to the realms of uncertainty and paradox that we're constantly buffered by, and this can only happen in a full-bodied, fullhearted way. It cannot be known; it can only be felt. Symbolic language is best suited to capture this universal challenge of being alone in our togetherness and feeling connected through our solitude. Or as Isabelle Robinet puts it: "The language of alchemy is a language that attempts to say the contradictory." This juggling and inversion of perspectives informs the nature of self and other; it's saying, "I exist because of you and you exist because of me" and extends this proclamation to all things.

We exist as people only through our relationships. Therefore, self-isolation is such a powerful experience. It can be torturous in the case of solitary confinement but also highly blissful and illuminating in the case of a meditation retreat. Our initial growth as humans, however, can't happen in isolation. We're entirely dependent on our parents and caregivers: self-regulation stems from co-regulation.[9]

As Barrett would suggest, we're also learning the cultural flavors and expressive movements of each emotion. And because our emotional learning is entangled with interoception—the felt sense of the body—

this means we're not only learning emotions from those around us but also how to inhabit our bodies. Our emotional granularity gradually crystallizes alongside our patterns of embodiment. This process never stops; however, we may seem to rigidify into our stories and structures of self-belief, but our identity is constantly being reinforced by those around us. Our neuroplasticity tapers off in our teenage years, but it never stops. We can learn, like the Daoists say, to breathe and become as a newborn.

This is why traveling and meeting new people can be such a transformative experience, as we naturally switch on our beginner's mind. It also explains how we often fail to notice how much change and growth can occur within a continuous familial relationship. It is also for this reason why people intentionally isolate themselves for spiritual transformation, as this cuts us off from our social circle's tendency to reinforce old patterns of identity.

We might stop here and frame our sense of embodiment and emotion as a product of our personal biology mixed alongside our social conditioning. However, our health and social nature are also embedded and entwined with the natural environment and all the life-forms we live in community with. We wouldn't exist without trees, water, sunlight, and food. Our relationality extends out from the human social sphere into the realms of animal, insect, plant, fungus, microbe, and mineral. We are in co-regulation with the nonhuman world, too.

This is where I have a more expansive view of emotion and consciousness as compared to most neuroscientists, for our emotional responses are not isolated to humans but happen also in relation to the natural world in which we are embedded. Who's to say that when I rejoice in jumping into the waves of the ocean that the ocean isn't also rejoicing with me? This harkens back to Chuang Tzu's famous parables of being able to know the delight of a river fish or questioning, after having dreamed of being a butterfly, whether he himself is within the dreamtime of a butterfly. Whereas we can frame dissociation as being on one point within the spectrum of human consciousness, there is also a wider multiplicity of consciousnesses that we are located within.

This is where the hidden value of dissociation lies, for it carries us beyond our skin and beyond our individualized and humanistic embodiment. This expansion of our embodied selves creates a sense of being embedded within a larger whole. Embeddedment reflects not only an intellectual appreciation for our interconnectedness with honeybees or oak trees, but it also creates a felt sense of being human, honeybee, and oak tree all at the same time.

It's no secret that from a modern psychiatric perspective most shamans would be considered psychotic and mentally deranged, as would many people experiencing a spiritually transformative experience. This is partly because the ability to extend our personhood into the world is extremely threatening to the ideals of the sovereign individual that modern culture is built upon. This is also partly why the phenomenon of dissociation has received so little attention by clinical researchers. It's not only hard to measure a disembodied experience, but for most scientists it's very difficult to believe or make sense of someone feeling as if they are outside their body and looking down on it, let alone accounts of astral travel or remote viewing.

Although most scientists disregard the mystical, it can't be ignored that many people who experience being dissociated or disembodied report that it can transform one's entire orientation in the world. Following is how Timothy Beardsworth describes a happenstance experience of this phenomenon.

> It was a beautiful sunny day, and I began looking at the hills which I could see from my window. What followed is almost impossible to express in words, but my whole mode of perception and my whole being suddenly altered. For what I think was a brief instant, though it seemed to last for a long time, I seemed to be "at one" with the hills, to be identified with them, to belong to them. My whole being was

absorbed in this feeling, which was of great intensity. . . . Then the "focus" altered, and I was looking at the hills normally again but feeling very startled at what had happened. I puzzled over it for weeks.[10]

Within Tibetan culture there has been an unparalleled exploration and dissemination of non-ordinary states of consciousness; following is Mingyur Rinpoche's account of an awakening experience.

As a drop of water placed in the ocean becomes indistinct, boundless, unrecognisable, and yet still exists, so my mind merged with space. It was no longer a matter of 'me' seeing trees, as I had become trees. Me and trees were one. . . . It seemed as if I could see forever, as if I could see through trees; as if I could be trees. I cannot even say I continued to breathe; Or my heart continued to beat. . . . There was no individual anything, no dualistic perception. No body, no mind, only consciousness. The cup that had contained empty space had broken, the vase had shattered, extinguishing "inside" and "outside". Through meditation I had known child luminosity, but never had I known such intense union of child and mother luminosity— emptiness infusing emptiness, the bliss of love and tranquility.[11]

Embeddedment is a little like the artistic technique of *sfumato* (the smoky blurring of edges), in this case between the boundary of our skin and the world around us. Embeddedment reflects something that is both experientially and scientifically known to be true: our personhood is a coming together of the brain, body, and environment.[12] Rather than see our personhood as merely a product of our brain, or the product of our brain-body, we can recognize our inter-being with our environment in a rational, reflective, and immediate sense. There is part of us that can appreciate the Earth as a part of our extended body. This is hinted at by Heidegger when he says, "I am my body, but I am also the space where my body is."

198 🌼 EMBODIMENT & DISEMBODIMENT

The philosopher of consciousness Bernardo Kastrup explains this conundrum well. He makes a strong argument that consciousness, not physical stuff, is the fundamental basis of the world. Rather than relying on intuition, he uses impeccable logic backed up by the most up-to-date scientific evidence to reach this conclusion.[13] His work is worth exploring in detail for those interested, but for our purpose I would point out one interesting detail that lies at the heart of his argument: he states that the phenomenon of dissociation is crucial evidence for understanding the nature of consciousness.

We now have hard proof that the human mind is capable of splitting into multiple selves. For years many scientists disbelieved that what was historically known as multiple personality disorder, and is now known as dissociative identity disorder (DID), even possible; they thought that patients were making it all up. But there is now clear evidence that one body can contain multiple minds, which are referred to as *alters*. The most striking evidence shows how one alter that claims and seems to be blind actually has a brain that switches off its physiological basis for vision, while another alter can switch it back on. This is something that is impossible to simply make up. What Bernardo extrapolates from this is that consciousness can dissociate from itself; it can split in two. He claims that our personal consciousness is a naturally occurring form of dissociation and that we are split off from what he calls mind-at-large.

In the same way that our senses have evolved with a bias toward survival over truth, this primordial dissociation is akin to what many of the great spiritual traditions point to—the self as illusion, the world as illusionary. Although this is an entirely natural part of life and allows us to individualize, it obscures a more truthful apprehension of consciousness as a universal phenomenon that co-arises among all things.

The co-arising nature of consciousness is not something experienced only by mystics and madmen. Within the social realm, this merging of self and other is termed *communitas* and happens within the spontaneity of music, dance, sport, and the ritual and trance traditions of religion and indigenous spirituality. Whereas from a medical lens this might be called a splitting away from self, it could equally be seen as simply expanding self. The work of Cranz and Illich might suggest that our more natural state is toward an ecological communitas, a natural sense of already being embedded within the world. This is very much aligned with the indigenous relationship with nature, of being in familiar kinship with all the shared life-forms of our habitat. Following is how the renowned anthropologist and primatologist Sarah Hrdy describes this relationship.

> What is striking about the worldview of foragers (among peoples as widely dispersed as the Mbuti of Central Africa, Nayaka foragers of South India, the Batek of Malaysia, Australian Aborigines, and the North American Cree) is that they tend to share a view of their physical environment as a giving place occupied by others who are also liable to be well-disposed and generous. They view their physical world as being in line with benevolent social relationships. Thus, the Mbuti refer to the forest as a place that gives, "food, shelter, and clothing just like their parents." The Nayaka simply say, "The forest is as a parent."[14]

This process of expanding into kinship with the world could be called the positive aspect of dissociation. It's not a threat to or fragmentation of our identity but rather a coming home to a grander sense of being. Dissociation certainly has many negative and unpleasant features, too. It can be framed a pathological disconnection from our felt sense of the body, and this happens frequently in response to a traumatic event, in the aftermath of trauma, or as a poorly understood brain disfunction. It can feel like a dreamy state, which can be confused with spiritual experiences and lead to spiritual bypass. In time, it can become a comfortable response to overwhelm, for it dulls the pain of existence. Unfortunately, it can also numb us to the magnificence and tangible bliss of life. Dissociation can also be infused with a subtle or intense fear and feel like being frozen or trapped.

In extreme cases, the sense of disconnection is felt not only from the physical body but also from our normal sense of self, creating fragmented selves that are compartmentalized from each other, as if we have a normal sense of self when we are functioning well and a different identity that responds to our memory of trauma. In extreme situations, this rupture of our identity can cause our minds to compartmentalize these different identities, as in dissociative identity disorder. The clinical experience and insight of Nijenhuis makes a clear case that DID is rooted in developmental trauma.

Although this might seem like an extreme phenomenon, the same process is occurring within most normal people, just at a lesser degree of intensity. We all have many masks as to who we are. Dissociation is extremely common in our society, and there isn't a clear differentiation between what is daydreaming for one person and what is pathological for another. Unfortunately, dissociation has a stigmatization in society. From outside observation, it might seem as if someone is acting strangely or is emotionally unresponsive. Their face might appear blank, or it could seem as if someone is glazed over or very clumsy. This is a shortsighted way to see this, though, as dissociation is most often an involuntary response to being physically or emotionally threatened.

There is also a self-stigmatization that happens, as often trauma is wrapped up in shame and self-disgust. Accompanying symptoms like dissociation create additional layers of emotion and self-judgment. Whether we face these symptoms in ourselves or in another, the challenge is to perceive each other with a greater depth of perception so that we can see beyond superficial appearances and masks.

This is indeed a challenge, for seeing dissociation in another can easily hijack our own social engagement system, making us believe we are being snubbed or emotionally dismissed. This can set off volatile chain reactions. It is socially taboo to be unresponsive in our facial or vocal expression—it can easily be interpreted as rude or aggressive. However, there is rarely such intention. Rather, dissociation is a protective biological response. Becoming numb protects us from pain, whether physical or emotional. It is extremely useful in a life-threatening situation but becomes a devastating crutch if it turns into a habitual response to stress.

The classic example is of the Scottish explorer David Livingstone, who while in Central Africa was attacked and mauled by a lion. His account of this experience is that upon being gripped and shaken by the jaws of the lion, his body went completely limp, and he felt as if he were looking down on the scene from outside his body. This numbed him to the full pain and horror of the situation. This experience of playing dead is not just a ploy but a state that our nervous system can go into involuntarily when in life-and-death situations. This happens in all mammals, as it gives us a last-ditch chance at survival.* It can also effectively numb the body through the release of endorphins, our highly potent natural painkillers.

Unfortunately, we humans have the tendency to use this response even when our perceived threat doesn't match the actual situation. More often than not, we are being cued by the internal sensations within our nervous system rather than external signs of danger. This is most readily seen in people with PTSD but is common to some degree in most people. If someone seems vacant, distracted, or not quite present, often they are disconnected from feeling their body. By reframing dissociation as a protective response to overwhelm, we can stop reinforcing self-judging and shameful emotions about our bodies and behavior. We can also learn to be more patient and compassionate to our spaced-out or unsociable friends and family.

We can see now that dissociation is a normal part of life and of our shared biology. And so how have other cultures responded to this

---

*This is because predators have their own survival instinct of being suspicious or disinterested in dead meat that might be contaminated; most are not scavengers.

phenomenon? In all traditional and premodern cultures there has been a historical tendency to view the effects of dissociation, trauma, and DID as some kind of possession. As the great writer Roberto Calasso describes:

> Ecstasy and possession are words that carry positive or negative connotations according to place and time. Both indicate metamorphic knowledge, the knowledge that transforms the person who knows at the moment at which he knows. The common assumption: a permeable mind, subject to the ebb and flow of elements that may at first sight seem extraneous but are also capable of establishing themselves as permanent guests. Yet where there is an I that is equipped with watertight compartments and is the supposed master of its own boundaries, ecstasy and possession can no longer enter. At the same time, the area that is knowable—or merely open to investigation—is vastly restricted.[15]

Even in modern times, the uncanniness of meeting someone who seems to have different identities, or an obscured, vacant identity, makes a strong impression. It's easy to see how most people throughout history interpret psychiatric issues as possession. There is also the cultural momentum to this narrative, which in the West has become completely delegitimized as superstitious and pagan. The scientific debunking of ghosts and spirits on top of the extremely negative view from Christian priests means that the concept of possession is doubly detested. Exorcism is viewed with cynicism and ridicule, whereas we are still none the wiser when it comes to what is actually happening in dissociation and DID. Trauma gives us a *why,* but we're still in the dark as to the *what* and *how* of dissociation. We simply have no scientific explanation for how consciousness can split from the body or fragment the identity.

In all shamanic cultures there's the tendency to see illness as an invasion of the body, the healing of which happens by dislodging, ameliorating, pulling, or sucking out the invading force. Chinese medicine developed in dialogue with these truly ancient shamanic practices, and so the first theoretical models of disease were seen as the body being invaded by different kinds of wind. The ancient classics of Chinese medicine say that "wind is the spearhead of the hundred diseases." This view evolved out of seeing the body as being invaded by evil forces. However, Chinese medicine from the start was framed within symbolic language, and so, we miss the point if we interpret this only as literal. Rather, the concept of wind could refer to multiple processes, and in its broadest sense to any kind of change. How we respond to the winds of change determines both our health and our fate. Disease arises from the inability to change. Layered on to this, the actual weather of wind was seen to carry disease into the body. Wind was seen as a universal breath, both in an environmental, personal, and cosmic sense. The internal space of the body was seen as a reflection of the external space of the natural environment; there's a continuum between the two, which was seen to resonate in specific patterns. And so, the internal winds of the body were seen as manifesting in emotion. The directionality of these winds determined whether we were in harmony with the greater patterns of growth and regeneration in nature.

This is how both physical and mental illness were initially explained—as a response to external pathogenic factors, which are symbolized by the words *wind, cold, heat,* and *dampness,* or to internal pathogenic factors, which are the emotions. As Chinese medicine evolved, it was influenced by different schools of thought, some with a more Confucianist perspective, some with a more Daoist or Buddhist. However, underneath the various models of classifying emotions and the patterns of nature, there was an undercurrent of practitioners who still engaged in exorcism and shamanic interventions. These practitioners were termed *fang-shi* and were generally in contrast to scholar-doctors. Whereas the more scholarly tradition would label acupuncture points as clearing heat or wind, the fang-shi would use these same points to clear someone of possession. They were known as ghost points, many of which happen to be located on the head and face.

In East Asian cultures, Daoism and Buddhism generally created a more holistic approach to nature, one that sought harmony with rather than dominion over the natural landscape. There was an overt blossoming of what may be called nondual consciousness, and this led to a less rigidified sense of the individual and a more malleable sense of personhood. In Buddhism, Daoism, and Vedanta, the fundamental ideas of identity and personhood were concluded to be illusory. We are an amalgam of selves, a Ponzi scheme of emotions, beliefs, and self-deceptions, and don't exist in any permanent unchanging way. Because of this, possession was not seen in a purely negative light but could harbor both blessing and curse.

Even to this day, there are many trance mediums who invite deities and spirit beings into their bodies, usually to impart spiritual insight, wisdom, and blessings or to act as oracles. The anthropologist Wade Davis says how in West Africa "spirit possession is the hand of divine grace . . . a very powerful transformative technique of ecstasy."[16] And if we look at the founders of most of the Daoist sects, we find that they all experienced some kind of trance mediumship or dream visitation from spirit beings or deities, and this is what actually initiated the sect or lineage. Even the modern art of tai chi was said to be imparted to Chang San Feng in a dream visitation by a mysterious immortal called Xuan Wu, the Dark Warrior. Just like in shamanic vision questing, we find that in Asia, dissociation and possession were a key feature in traditional spirituality.

The question then arises: Where is the distinction between these different types of possession? The traditional viewpoints vary greatly and are so alien to modern sensibilities that we need to again reflect that these viewpoints came from a symbolic, multidimensional stance. There is a close etymological link between the Chinese character for *ghost* (Gu) and for *parasite* (Gui). If we entertain the idea that we are embedded within a multiplicity of consciousnesses, then the idea that we could become possessed by bacterial, parasitic, or viral processes that inhabit both our microbiome and the organic environment becomes less far-fetched.

We know that the presence of certain types of bacteria or virus in our gut and body will influence not only our eating decisions and cravings but will also affect our health and behavior in countless ways. A fascinating example is the single-celled parasite called toxoplasma gondii, which is estimated to be harbored by a third of the global population and is linked to an increased risk of neuroticism and suicide. If we consider that our vagus nerve is intricately involved in regulating our microbiome, this brings another dimension to how vagal tone is involved in both emotional regulation and conducting the shifting porosity in our embodiment and personhood. This is potentially why the Daoist practices yield more insight into this phenomenon, as they place more emphasis on working with the abdominal space and the material aspects of embodiment than the mind-only schools of Buddhism and Vedanta.

In our modern age, we are plagued with addiction and an insatiable consumerism that has spawned the emergence of the attention economy. We are as equally prone to mind viruses and memetic malware as we are to real viruses and infectious disease. In both cases, I believe it's helpful to expand our notions of dissociation and possession beyond the negative connotations they possess. Instead, we can reframe ourselves as living within an ecology of consciousness and information. By this, I mean that our individual sovereignty is never watertight but always in relationship and transformation through the air we breathe, the people with whom we share space, and all the unknown processes we are embedded within.

This is the natural state of life; purity of self is only an illusion. It's good to sometimes remember that we're composed of dead and reconstituted plant life, mostly. Nevertheless, we can strike a right balance, a right relationship to where we stand within this ecology of being.

This starts by recognizing ourselves in other people, in other life-forms around us, and surrendering to a give-and-take reciprocity between our personal interiority and external world. Counterintuitively, this openness to the world allows us to feel more at home within ourselves. What we relinquish of our control, and of our old sense of self, we gain in the freedom of discovering a new story of interrelationship with the world.

In this light, both traditional acupuncture points and Dien Chan can be used to help us clear our mind and body of unhelpful types of possession. They can be used to counter dissociation and come home to a sense of belonging in our bodies and place of living.

It's interesting to note that nearly every acupuncture point on the head and face has the primary function of clearing either wind or heat. The sense portals are gateways to possession, and the points surrounding the senses can be used to release what we're possessed by, whether it is an emotion, idea, infection, ghost, or mind virus. In many ways, the nasal cavity, eyes, and throat are the immune system's first line of defense; therefore, opening and clearing our senses is an important preventive measure on many levels. The next Dien Chan sequences we'll explore open the lymphatic circulation and energetic pathways of the neck and face. They also activate many of the spirit points that are traditionally used to clear our mind and reclaim our embodiment.

FOURTEEN

· ·

Dien Chan
for Embodiment
& Homecoming

Form is Emptiness, Emptiness is Form.

THE PRAJNAPARAMITA HEART SUTRA

Using Dien Chan to counteract the effects of trauma is a nuanced and multilayered endeavor. As we've explored, the language of trauma can box in our conceptions of what's normal or abnormal, whereas different cultures interpret and address the same phenomenon in different ways. There's a fine balance between the normalization of pathological habits of embodiment and perception and the tendency to interpret everything in life as a symptom of one's trauma.

It's helpful to remember the saying "Normal people are simply people we haven't got to know yet." There are many aspects of our health that are entirely outside measurement, classification, or quantification. Given the cultural differences in the understanding of trauma, perhaps we can shift our interpretation of dissociation, anxiety, shame, or overwhelm so that it isn't framed purely as a negative symptom of illness.

207

Rather, we can see these sensations as a natural response to the hardship life presents us. In this light, we can begin reframing these sensations. Specifically, we can begin to see how difficult emotions and sensations are often a defense response rather than a sign of brokenness or decrepitude. This presents us with breathing space and the choice to let go of self-judgment and blame, thus opening a path toward working with the body's natural intelligence and capacity for healing. The sign this is happening is an increased connection to our felt sense of the body and the gradual ability to feel safe in our heart.

There are two self-care techniques that follow. One is very simple and quick; the other includes a sequence of steps. Both can be used to increase our sense of embodiment and feeling at home in our selves.

✿ A Point Technique for Grounding and Revival

This technique is famous throughout Chinese medicine and folk practice and has been used to revive countless people after fainting or losing consciousness. It's also a go-to point for epileptic seizures and strokes. Even though these are extreme cases, this technique can also be used to revive ourselves if we feel dissociated, fatigued, or unalert.

The technique is simply to either press or pinch the acupuncture point known as Du26/*Ren Zhong*/Central Being, which overlaps with the Dien Chan point 63. This point lies in the hollow space above the upper lip, known as the philtrum (see figure 11.2, step 7, part 1, on page 166). We can use the thumb and forefinger to squeeze the whole philtrum, holding for a few seconds at a moderate strength. Or we can use a fingertip or knuckle to press the point slowly but firmly.

Point 63 is often intuitively tapped when we need to compose our thoughts. It can be an easy on-the-go point to help compose and ground ourselves. Although it seems very simple, there is a deep, esoteric secret behind this point. To understand this, we must look to the name. In English, the word *philtrum* stems from the

Greek *phil*—"to love"—and *trum*—"charm or talisman". The philtrum embodies the charm of eros; it draws us back to the world. There was an innate knowing that this part of our body relates to both the erotic as well as the more cosmic dimensions of love—what is called *agape* in Greek, "universal love".

If we think about it afresh, the philtrum is indeed a curious aspect of the face; it's sensuous and bridges the space between taste, breath, and aroma. In the Jewish tradition there is a very old folk story about the philtrum holding the secret to our humanity and that before we were born every human is touched by an angel on this point, which acts as amnesia to this secret. This was also apprehended by the ancient Chinese, who named the philtrum *Ren Zhong,* which translates as "Human Center" or "Central Being" (Du26). Love is central to humanity; when we touch this point, it can remind us of this secret.

The way the Chinese concealed this secret is through a type of cosmo-eroticism, a language describing the interplay between Heaven and Earth. Through a symbolic lens, when an ancient Chinese seer beholds a human face, there is the recognition of a similar pattern between the appearance of the human face and the Yi Jing's eleventh hexagram, known as Tai (Great Peace). The paired orifices of the ears, eyes, and nostrils form the three upper yin lines, while the mouth and two lower orifices form the three lower, single yang lines. This hexagram consists of Earth above Heaven, and the interplay between them creates humanity—the human in the center, between Heaven and Earth.

Although to someone unfamiliar with the Yi Jing this might all seem obscure, the significance of this hexagram is highly relevant to Chinese medicine. In a way, it illustrates the whole rationale for healthy living. The renowned healer and Classical Chinese Medicine teacher Liu Lihong describes this clearly.

If we were to describe life in terms of normal and abnormal circumstances, the best description might be the contrast between the hexagrams Tai and Pi. Pi represents the state in which health and vitality are lost; it is also the state of disease. Tai, on the other hand, obviously represents a state of health and prosperity. From a Chinese Medicine perspective, one of the chief goals of medicine is to convert the state represented by Pi to the state represented by Tai.[1]

Because of this, the Du26/*Ren Zhong*/Central Being acupoint, which is at the juncture of the two central channels of the body, is used to resuscitate life—it has a unique ability to call the spirit back into the body. This is also reflected in Dien Chan, which calls this point Major Yang and considers it perhaps the most important point after point 0. In both Dien Chan and Chinese medicine this point's function is to revive yang, literally bringing us back to life. In terms of the embodiment of the face, this point has a centering effect. It has a holographic resonance with our Dan Tien, our whole body center, and can bring us into resonance with the cosmological yang energy—the source of creativity and inspiration. This Zhong Qi, or central vitality, inspires the natural restorative power of the body.

❀ Self-Care Sequence for Embodiment and Immunity

This sequence works on many levels—it reconnects our head with our body; it increases the lymphatic circulation, which helps clear our sinuses and fortify our immune system. It's particularly good for releasing tension from the neck and thereby increasing the pathways of communication between the head and body, allowing us to more easily drop our awareness and come to rest in the base of our body. It also engages many of the acupuncture points known as the Windows of the Sky and the Thirteen Ghost Points, which are specifically used to clear the senses, increase our tranquillity and connection to the sacred, and as a mode of soul retrieval. As such, if we choose, we can bring the intention of clearing our senses, mind, and body of any type of possession, whether it's viral, technological, memetic, or spiritual.

1. Cross your arms and use the palms to gently grasp and release the biceps and upper arms for ten seconds.

2. Keep your arms crossed and used cupped palms to gently pat over each collarbone. Do this for ten seconds on each side.

3. Uncross the arms and use the fingers to gentle pat into the space just above each collarbone, working in and out horizontally for ten seconds.

4. Use the thumb and knuckle of the forefinger to gentle squeeze and pull up and down the sternocleidomastoid muscles (the big V muscles at the front of the neck) for ten seconds (see figure 14.1).

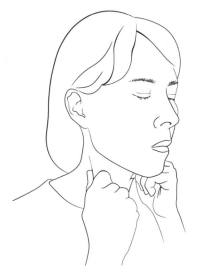

Figure 14.1. Self-Care for Embodiment and Immunity
Step 4, massaging down the sternocleidomastoid muscle. This step gently releases the ST9/*Ren Ying*/ People Welcome acupuncture point.

5. Use the first three fingers as hooks to press and slide down the area behind the ears, under the bone. Work horizontally along the occiput (back ridge of the skull) toward the back of the neck for ten seconds.

6. Make scissor hands and press and slide the fingers on either side of the ears. Gently open and close the jaw to open this space between the ears, face, and head. Do this for ten seconds.

7. Use the fingers to circle-rub over the temples for five to ten seconds.

8. Use the index fingertips to rub the areas between the inside corners of the eyes and the bridge of the nose for five to ten seconds.

9. Gently sweep the fingertips over the eyelids, upper eyes, and lower eyes, as if you're sweeping dust out of your eyes, for five to ten seconds.

10. Use the knuckles to sweep outward from the center of the forehead toward the temples, working out the whole forehead this way for five to ten seconds.

11. Use the ridge of the index finger knuckle to sweep under the cheekbones, then use the points of the knuckles to press down over the masseter muscle (the chewing muscle) for five to ten seconds.

12. Use the ridge of the index knuckles of each hand—one to press the nose to the side, the other to cause traction by pressing the eyebrow to the other side. Hold for a breath, then switch sides. Use this same traction force by pressing the bridge of the nose downward while pressing the third-eye area upward (see figure 14.2).

13. Use the fingertips to press alongside the chin while the thumbs press up underneath the jawbone, into the base of the lower pallets, working outward toward the ears for five to ten seconds.

14. Sweep the hands over the face, downward and away, as if clearing any tension off the brow and face.

15. Repeat step 6, using scissor hands to open the jaw.

16. Repeat step 5, opening the base of the neck.

17. Repeat step 4, working down the sternocleidomastoid muscle.

18. Repeat step 2, patting cupped hands over the collarbones and chest.

19. Finish by combing the hands down the neck, arms, and rib cage, as well as across the chest.

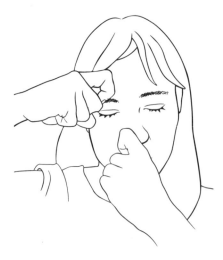

Figure 14.2. Self-Care for Embodiment and Immunity Step 12, creating traction between the nose and brow to release the sinuses.

This sequence is great to use if you're feeling fuzzy headed or congested. It can facilitate the clearing of the sinuses and so you may find yourself needing to blow your nose afterward. Because we're essentially renewing the lymphatic circulation of the face, this sequence is helpful to use before traveling into any large crowd of people, such as at airports or on subways. It will buffer up the first layer of our immune system, where our boundary with the world is most porous and accessible. It's also for this reason that we initially open the pathways between the neck and head, for this opens the flow of circulation to then release the face and sinuses.

The aftereffect of this sequence doesn't only help us feel clearheaded physically, but it makes it easier to drop down from our heads and feel at home in the body. The tension we hold in our neck is both involved in the postural feat of balancing the heavy weight of our heads upon our spine as well as the bracing of our embodied selves within the structure of the skull. This often correlates with what is called the sympathetic dominance of the nervous system, which activates our senses to be on high alert. Even though the senses become highly focused on risk and danger, they can actually lose the big picture, losing the "forest for the trees," as they say. We lose our contentment and belonging when we're faced with continuous danger; therefore, by using this sequence to come into touch with our parasympathetic (vagal) nervous system, we shift into a more balanced way of being in the world. We also thereby switch on our social nervous system, which opens us to dialogue, listening, and positive social engagement.

Interestingly, one of the main Window of Heaven points is right at the midpoint between the face and the heart, just to the side of the Adam's apple, and the age-old name for this point is *Ren Ying,* which means "People Welcome" (ST9). This reflects how our social nervous system and vagus nerve, which connects through this area between the face and heart, was apprehended by Chinese acupuncturists more than two thousand years ago. This point was needled to help with the psychological tendency of feeling anti-social, timid, and untrusting of other people. Feeling relaxed and open from this area of our throat allows us to welcome the presence of other people.

This sequnce also frees our voice, enabling us to speak from our heart and connect to other people. Feeling comfortable and at home within our own skin helps us form relationships. Our capacity for relationship, to form strong and deep bonds with the world and with other beings, is the measure of true wealth and health. If we have all the money and perfect health but not a friend in the world, we won't feel rich or have well-being. But if we can feel comfortable in our body and secure in our relationships, this builds the basis for both our health and for exploring the full depths of our connection with the world.

Belonging and contentment precipitate a feeling of safety in the present moment. Safety opens a gateway to curiosity. When we're curious, this pauses all animosity and allows us to connect with others. Curiosity also forms a bridge into wonder, awe, and revery. It extends our capacity to relate with the otherness and strangeness of life. Or, as David Bentley Hart says, "The sudden awareness that no mere fact can possibly be an adequate explanation of the mystery in which one finds oneself immersed in at every moment." These feelings and callings catalyze our innate creativity, giving birth to new ideas and forging new pathways.

This is where Dien Chan, qigong, and meditation can come into a unique harmony, for they can elicit a transformation of our senses, enabling us to change our embodiment and perception. When we look and listen with curiosity, awe, and wonder, we can start to see beyond the appearances of things and acquire a greater depth in our capacity to relate to the world. Not only does this shift old patterns of thinking and behavior, but it heightens our ability to savor the delights and deliciousness of the world as well.

FIFTEEN

● ●

Returning to Our Senses

*The real voyage of discovery consists not of seeking new
landscapes but in seeing with new eyes.*

MARCEL PROUST

In this book we have explored how Dien Chan can be used for improving our health, embodiment, and well-being. In essence, this process begins with increasing our ability to feel in to our body and learning to develop a sense of calmness and safety conjoined with an inquisitive curiosity. Feeling safe in our bodies is the first step toward healing the effects of chronic stress and trauma.

Being able to maintain this sense of calm curiosity during the arousal of emotion plays an important part in re-patterning our nervous systems and renewing our health and vitality. The face can act in this respect as a bridge into safety—it is both a reservoir of emotion and a catalyst for its release. And so, Dien Chan offers us a way to untangle and reset our emotional dynamics, which in turn affects our overall health in many ways.

There is another dimension to this process that's important to recognize, which we'll explore in these final chapters, beginning with acknowledging that both the layers of tension and the habitual expressions of our face are intimately linked to the idea of who we are. The face is an embodied symbol of our whole life, of all the stories that make up our identity and character. In turn, our mental-emotional template shapes how we see, hear, and interact with the world and people around us.

Dien Chan offers us a tool to both change our patterns of identity and perform a type of alchemy of perception. When we release the facial tension and habitual microexpressions that surround our eyes, ears, nose, and mouth, our sensitivity to the world changes. Our attention widens beyond threat perception. This opens a heightened ability to savor and delight and to find wonderment in what was previously mundane. Dien Chan affords us a window of opportunity to change our emotional expression and how we perceive ourselves and others. This alchemy of perception not only changes the appearance of the world in the unfolding present moment but can also transmute the story of who we are. The past can be revealed in a new light.

When we experience a major disruption in our personal narrative, such as a tragedy or trauma, the stories we tell ourselves about who we are can stop making sense. This happens both cognitively and viscerally and, therefore, can feel like both a psychological crisis and a disjunction within our body and nervous system. In psychotherapy this is termed a dysregulation of the nervous system.

The challenge of healing requires that we envision ourselves within a new story rather than simply reconfiguring ourselves within the old one. Healing is not about returning to who we were before trauma but about entering a new chapter in our story. It is not about returning to a pre-tragic version of ourselves but to coming into a post-tragic way of being. As Einstein famously stated, "Problems cannot be solved with the same mind-set that created them."

Instead, we must discover new ways of thinking and new ways of being in our bodies. And this begins by feeling the newness of our body in each present moment. Increasing our vagal tone and the ability to feel more deeply and be mindful of our body is crucial to healing a dys-regulated nervous system.

Dien Chan can bring us in touch with the energetic charge and intimacy of our stories as they manifest in the face. If we can find the right kind of touch, then we can unmask ourselves from those stories that no longer serve us. If we can maintain a sense of calmness, safety, and curiosity, Dien Chan can pinpoint the somatic dimension of self-deception.

Many of the stories we tell ourselves about ourselves are not absolutely true but instead are creative deceptions. Sometimes this is quite helpful, as it allows us to function in the world. However, if we are honest with ourselves, the story of our identity plays a major role in all the suffering, anguish, and poor health we experience.

Seeing ourselves as something that we're not, or wishing ourselves to be different from who we truly are, can cause no end of suffering. And all these emotional patterns and masks that surround our self-value are mirrored by the physical contractions of the muscles and tissues in our face. Physical, mental, and emotional are intertwined.

Therefore, Dien Chan can be used to engage and question these habitual contractions in our expression and identity. It allows us to explore the masks that we wear. Crucially, if we can amplify our inner curiosity then we can increase our felt sense of personhood as it is embodied through our face. Or, in other words, staying with the feelings in our face can help unveil our masks and self-deceptions.

This reveals something remarkable: even though our face can assume the form of a mask—that is, a fixed and unchanging expression—if we pay close attention, we'll notice our face is ever-changing. This small act of recognition gifts us with this valuable piece of self-knowledge: our personhood is in a continual state of redefinition. We're all making it up as we go along! In ten year's time, you will be a different person according to how you creatively redefine yourself through each present moment.

We can change, and, as Rilke says, we must change. This natural spontaneity flies in the face of the notion that we have a fixed and permanent identity. Life is improvisational, there is always something unexpected going on, whether or not we are aware of it. When our face responds to the world with the freedom of spontaneity, we move toward experiencing our original face. Getting stuck in a mask, or in a role or pantomime we believe so strongly in, can take us out of resonance with the natural spontaneity and regenerative capacity of nature.

The notion that we wear masks is fairly easy to grasp in that we all instinctively get into character to suit different occasions. Our perception also overlays masks upon other peoples' faces. A useful adage illustrates this: "Whenever two people meet, there are always six people present. There is each man as he sees himself, each man as the other person sees him, and each person as they really are."

But how do we get past the masks and see one another beyond pretensions and masquerades? This is surely where true dialogue and connection happens. However, the idea that we can take off all our masks and unveil an original face is a little mischievous and riddle-like in itself. It begs the question: What is my authentic self? Who am I at my most bare-naked level?

There is both mystery and paradox here. For we can answer these questions superficially, by defining ourselves by our parts—our appearance, name, family, and personal history. But we are more than the sum of our parts. The analytical mind or the anatomical body will never comprehend the whole person. This way of knowing will always draw a dividing line that separates us from our full interconnectivity.

Historically, this is where the notion of the soul comes in, that we have some kind of atomistic essence that defines our innermost being. But in modern times this explanation has lost its prescience, for both our consciousness and identity are popularly explained as resulting simply from the brain-body dynamic. In either case, both views are susceptible to this overly analytic way of thinking. In Buddhist and Daoist culture, and in the more recent cognitive science, there is the premise that our personhood is the result of brain, body, and environment.* Like Indra's Net of Jewels, there is a co-arising and interdependence among all things.

This is a key understanding that is directly experienced through qigong practice and is at the heart of Classical Chinese Medicine—that our identity is not defined purely by our embodiment. We are not only the result of our brain and body. We are also continuously resulting anew, in a state of becoming, and this is by virtue of our dialogue and participation with the world around us. The relational nature of our personhood is not limited to our social circles but is instead enmeshed in the wider nonhuman orbits we're held within.

What I have termed *embeddedment* reflects this experience—true embodiment doesn't divide us from the world outside our bodies but allows us to feel the becoming of the world through our bodies. Our individuality is never truly closed off from others. Rather, we are like an open whole. And we can feel and partake in the regeneration and growing wholeness of nature through the openness of our face, heart, and belly. Our original face speaks to this implicit connection in which our personhood is embedded through everything we have known and touched, and yet is still emerging in new and unseen ways.

---

*The particular branch of cognitive science that advocates this is known as 4E Cog-Sci, which postulates that cognition isn't limited to the head but is also embodied, embedded, enacted, and extended. This is echoed in the clinical work of Ellert Nijenhuis, who in his concluding summary in *Trinity of Trauma,* states that "there is a trinity of the brain, the body, and the environment. That is, the brain, the body, and the environment are intrinsically related. The brain cannot exist without a (wider) body, the (wider) body not without a brain, and the brain-body not without a material and social environment. . . . Mind depends on the trinity of the brain, the body, and the environment, just as the concepts of the brain, the body, and the environment depend on experiencing and knowing minds. One implication is that the mind is not in the head." This carries one toward an understanding of consciousness that is all-pervasive, which is most clearly explained in the work of Bernardo Kastrup. It is important to note that this view does not contradict science but is actually more congruent and parsimonious with the current science. However, it does contradict the dogmatic opinions that the current paradigm holds as consensus.

This relational function of our being is mediated through the face and body. Our face is unique in this way because of the sense portals, which carry the light, sound, and aromas of the world into our body. Our eyes, ears, nose, and mouth enable a vivid participation and relationality with the world. Therefore, they play a vital role in the creation of our present self and who we might become. Dien Chan explores all the expressive and emotional patterns that surround and modulate our sense portals. It's this exploration of the face as a medium between inner and outer that can clear and open a new vision for our future and shed new light on our past, effectively transforming the old stories we usually hold as fixed. Or as John Moriarty says, "We have a new past to emerge from." When we enter different modes of perception, we can profoundly reorient the way we look at our lives.

This alchemy of perception begins at the physical level and progresses toward the more subtle, conscious, and energetic. Dien Chan specifically releases the physical tension and emotional contraction that is held around our sense organs. If we pay attention to this release, we can notice and encourage a parallel shift in our perception. This shift changes how we perceive the world around us but is also a shift in our self-perception and felt sense of the body.

This process has an interesting parallel with the cutting edge of stress and trauma therapy, which recognizes how our perception can be skewed when our nervous system is tightened into a threat response. We pay attention to the world in a very different way when our survival is at stake. Being always set to survival mode can be catastrophic, for we see each person we meet as a potential threat and are unconsciously scanning our environment for the worst possible outcomes; all beauty is drained from the world. This happens not only when we have unresolved trauma but also when we see the world purely through an analytic lens, or when emotions like anger overwhelm us.

If we're annoyed or angry, we can become completely blind to the delicious fragrances and beauty around us. We can lose the ability to savor and delight in the simplest pleasures, like the coolness of drinking fresh water or the sound of the wind in the trees. We all have layers of dissociative perception that blank out big swathes of life as normal or bland, when in reality we are continuously buffered by spectacular and outrageous things. The extraordinary is concealed within the ordinary, if we only pay attention.

By bringing attention to how our perception can modulate our body state, we can re-pattern our nervous system and mode of being in the world. There is intriguing evidence that therapies like EMDR (Eye Movement Desensitization and Reprocessing), which uses vision in novel ways, or Stephen Porges's Safe and Sound protocol, which uses hearing in novel ways, can create profound shifts in both our perception and the state of our nervous system and mind. They can bring us back to a feeling of safety in the body. At a bare-bones level, just the simple practice of orienting, of naming five things we can see, hear, touch, or smell, can be an effective way of soothing the nervous system, grounding the body, and turning down any alarms bells that are being triggered by our threat-detection system.

In a similar vein, the first step in using Dien Chan to change our perception is to return the senses to the body. This is most easily done when your surrounding environment is familiar, feels safe, and doesn't have any loud or disturbing sounds, sights, or aromas. The modern world has created a specter of hyperstimulation for our senses, and we must attempt to quiet the overload to which we have grown so accustomed. Bringing the senses home to the body is called inner hearing or inner vision in Daoist practice, as mentioned previously. It's closely akin to the inner touch of interoception—the felt sense of the body. Can we reverse our senses inward and behold all the rich and ever-flowing change inside us?

When we use techniques that combine Dien Chan with the Golden

Elixir practice, we can more effectively bring a sense of quietude and stillness to the felt sense of our mind-body. The sealing of our senses cuts out the clatter and turbulence the outside world presents to us; it turns down the volume and clears the wind and heat from our interiority. Once we can establish this darkening of the senses, which in the language of the Golden Elixir is called putting the lid on the cauldron, we can then return to the world with an increased sense of clarity and calmness. We can rest and reset our perception.

The longer we can maintain equanimity—that is, perceiving with as little grasping or pushing away as possible—the more we will be able to sense the world afresh. Not only is this a catalyst for inspiration and wonder, but it will lessen the emotional reactivity that occurs when we hear, see, touch, or smell something volatile.

Our vision, hearing, touch, taste, and smell can be changed by physically touching the sense organs. By decongesting and releasing both the physical and energetic stagnation around our eyes, ears, nose, and mouth, it becomes easier to relax the more subtle aspects of our perception. Fully relaxing our face, like a Buddha, opening the possibility of changing the stories that are linked to the mental and emotional contraction within our face and mind. The key to this process is to realize that the physical act of relaxation is a direct parallel of mental equanimity.

Relaxation can sometimes be experienced with a note of pushing away, turning away from, or dissociation. The whole idea of relaxation is overly associated with being stressed, which is why people generally do not like being told to relax. Usually this just serves to accuse someone of being stressed. Therefore, we must uncouple physical relaxation from any type of anti-stress prescription. There is no binary between being stressed and being relaxed. Instead, we might frame relaxation as a state of flow, or as a never-ending continuum of rest and bliss. Regardless, the type of relaxation that changes our embodiment involves staying present within our body as we let go.

In Zen meditation this process is sometimes called the backward step. To step backward from the superficiality of the face or our sense of fixed identity means to shift our awareness backward into the body—from the front toward the center and back of the head. By releasing the specific points and areas of contraction in our face, we can begin to feel our face and our personhood not as a conglomeration of parts but as a resonant whole.

Feeling our whole face, together as one, opens us to the wholeness in our body and in nature, creating a sense of spaciousness, giving fresh energy to the sensuous. The world becomes less and less tinged with our own stories and more vibrant and awake. We start to defy the old Talmudic saying that we see the world "not as it is but as we are." We come closer to the *suchness* of things when our curiosity verges off into wonder and awe.

John Moriarty calls this silver branch perception—to come to a vivid encounter with life in full disclosure.[1] He describes this way of perceiving as like "being raided by unearthly sweetness," to awaken to the world's implicit wonder and effervescence, and in the aftermath, a profound readjustment to one's immediate surroundings, a recognition that "all bushes are burning bushes, all ground is holy ground."

To see with new eyes, as Proust says, is not to literally have new eyes but to learn to see life in its ever-unfolding wonderment. However, the first step is to come back to the ordinary, noticing what we perceive as normal. This means noticing and being okay with the mundane in our lives, without any craving for extreme sensuality or excitement for stimulation. Again, these embodied gestures of the backward step and the downward flow anchor us from being swept up by excitement or agitation. The following practices offer guidance in this first step of quieting and resetting our senses. This is the groundwork that can develop calmness, deepen equanimity, and gradually open us to new feelings of wonder and awe.

DIEN CHAN MEDITATIONS FOR
RETREAT, SAFETY, AND PURIFICATION

❦ Sealing the Senses

1. Rub and warm the palms together, then close the eyes and press the palms over the eyes.
2. Raise the eyebrows so the outer edge of the palms presses into the eyeball.
3. Press and slide the palms over toward the ears and press onto the ears, sealing off sound.
4. Circle-rub the palms and then slowly sweep the hands down the sides of the neck.

This technique is often used instinctively when life becomes too much. The emotional impression of someone covering their eyes or ears is usually of someone overwhelmed. This shows us how intermeshed our perception is with emotion. Although this technique can be helpful whenever there's a feeling of sensory or emotional overstimulation, it can also be a powerful way of resetting our vision and hearing so we have more perceptual and emotional clarity.

❦ Tapping the Heavenly Drum

1. Place both palms over each ear so the fingers rest behind the head at the base of the skull. Make sure the palms cup the ears to block out any external noise. Likewise, close the eyes and turn your senses inward.
2. Very gently start to tap all the fingers, listening to the sounds created and feeling all the subtle tension release from the occiput, at the base of the skull. Continue for a few slow breaths.
3. After you release the hands and gently open the eyes, pay attention to the quality of your hearing and clarity of vision.

This technique has its origins in the Golden Elixir practice and carries a range of purposes. It increases our capacity to draw our senses inward, specifically into hearing the internal space within the head. The regions of the brain that are being stimulated correlate with our vision, as well as with the brain stem—the bridge between our spinal cord and brain. For this reason, it's recommended to practice this technique with the spine upright and aligned.

The main acupuncture points being stimulated are GB20/*Feng Chi*/Wind Pool, BL10/*Tian Zhu*/Celestial Pillar, and Du16/*Feng Fu*/Wind Palace. These points release and fortify against invasive forces and are used to soothe the mind, improve sleep, and ease headaches. This technique helps bring a sense of balance into our nervous system and also has a purifying and brightening effect on the senses.

🌸 Red Dragon Stirs the Ocean

1. Place the tip of the tongue on the upper palate, at the most sensitive point just behind the front teeth. Gently tap the teeth together nine times, at a slow pace of just under a second per tap. Listen to the internal sound created. After each tap, feel in to the jaw muscle and the lower palate, giving the intention to soften and release after each contraction. After the last tap, keep the tip of the tongue in place but fully relax the back of the throat, jaw, and lower palate.
3. Press the tip of the tongue into the left cheek and roll the tongue all the way over to the right cheek, circling in one direction three times, then the other direction three times. Then squeeze the tongue against the outside of the teeth and gums, again circling three times in both directions.
4. Feel any saliva that is generated and gently swallow it as if this is medicine, consciously feeling this sweet dew nourish the body all the way to the belly.

This technique is also a classic of Golden Elixir practice and seeks to increase our ability to be a nourishment unto ourselves. While saliva isn't usually given much thought, in qigong practice saliva can be transmuted from a digestive fluid into Divine Water or Sweet Dew, thought to aid not only in digestion but also in nourishing all aspects of our health and mind.

In many ways, good health rests on a foundation of healthy teeth and gums. Although mundane, keeping our teeth and gums healthy is a primary aspect of keeping our body healthy. As obvious as it sounds, it's good to remind ourselves why we all keep a daily regimen for keeping our teeth healthy. Not only is this a wonderful time to introduce mindfulness into daily life, but through extension we can reflect on the necessity of keeping our speech and language healthy, too. By consciously stretching our tongue and the muscles we use to form speech, we encourage clarity in our voice. On top of this, the root of the tongue extends all the way down to the heart. As such, it travels along a major thoroughfare of our vagus nerve. By stretching the tongue, we encourage vagal tone.

🪷 Thunder Skull Toning

1. Place the pads of each thumb so as to plug your ears, blocking out external noise. Close your eyes and rest the middle fingers atop your eyelids. The index, ring, and pinky can rest gently where they land on the face.

2. Take a very slow, deep breath into the belly, and on the exhale intone *Om*, with the emphasis on the resonant humming of the *mmmmmm*. Repeat three times, feeling your full attention absorbed in the resonant sound through the skull. As you release the hands, feel into the increased quietude created from the intonations.

This technique comes from Indian pranayama and is a wonderful and easy way to clear the head of thoughts and bring a sense of clarity to our hearing and vision. By blocking the external senses and feeling the strong vibration of the breath and voice within the body, we shift our attention inward, helping us develop our internal hearing.

The breath and voice are powerful tools for creating lasting change in our mind and body. The simple act of turning the vibration of the voice inward, instead of projecting the voice outward, has multiple effects. Like a personal sonic massage, we can release tension through the face, head, throat, and chest in this fashion. The out-breath specifically tones the vagus nerve, which is why a long outward sigh has a relaxing effect on the nervous system. This is also why the practice of singing has many hidden health benefits, for it opens our breathing capacity as well as increases vagal tone, especially when singing socially.

This technique is also helpful for vibrating open the sinuses. When we hum, we not only vibrate through the nasal and cranial cavity, but we also increase nitric oxide, which is an essential component for health and mental well-being.

As the notes from these practices suggest, there are multiple layers and benefits. On the one hand, there are some immediate tangible effects in down-regulating our nervous system and creating physiological changes in the tissues and fluids of the face and head. On the other hand, the more we engage in each exercise with a clear awareness, and with equanimity, the more we can modulate these effects through intention.

For our purposes, the intention is to bring home the senses and turn them around so that we don't send out our hearing, vision, or touch but keep them held within. There are two movements of awareness here.

One is the backward step, which is a shift of awareness from the surface of the face toward the center and back of the head. This backward shift brings our senses inward from the outer surface of each sense organ to the space just behind the eyes, ears, nose, and mouth. We begin to listen in to the space behind the eyes and feel the space within each inner ear.

The other movement is the downward flow, which is a coming in to touch with the heart and pelvic bowl. Instead of thinking that our sense perception is simply a mechanism that happens strictly between our eyes and brain, or the ears and the brain, this downward flow gives us a felt sense of how our chest, breath, organs, nervous system, and abdomen are also contingent for perception.

When we can bring both movements together, we can start to change our mode of perception. We are harnessing the power of the vagus nerve, the wisdom in our body, to make better sense of the world. The presence of our heart and belly changes our sense-making. Ideally, when we practice these techniques with the right intention, we'll start to feel calmer in our bodies, clearer in our head and senses, and more at ease and peaceful within our surroundings.

Once we feel comfortable with these practices and can create a slowing down and quieting effect on our mind-body, we can then return outward and engage our perception in a more active way. We can harness the imaginal in the way we look at others and orient in the world.

Before pursuing this, it's very helpful to create a stable foundation in the ordinariness of our bodies and senses, and so it's recommended to use the practices in this chapter both preliminarily and as way of staying grounded in the face of excitement or activation. This brings us to the next chapter, exploring the basis for wonder and delight.

SIXTEEN

Silver Branch Perception

If we need a vision that can open a future alternative to the one predetermined by our past, we have it: the silver branch. . . . The silver branch is a universal ontology, an epiphany come among us of what everything essentially and fundamentally is.

JOHN MORIARTY

Our senses are receptive to a phenomenal amount of information. It's estimated that in just one second, we can unconsciously register up to thirteen million bits of information. Of this staggering number, we're consciously aware of about fifty bits of information, which is still quite a lot if you consider how many colors, sounds, and smells you can pinpoint right now.[1] But, even though we have this incredibly fine-tuned sensory apparatus, in reality we're only perceiving the tiniest fraction of the informational richness of the world around us. This is why we invented telescopes and microscopes. It is also why we've evolved a mythical, symbolic, and imaginal perception, so that we might relate to the unseen patterns and import of the world to, "think around corners," as it were.*

We think of our perception as a truthful account of the world *out there*, but our brain and senses are more like filters that trim the world around us so we perceive only what's relevant for living. This is a metaphorical way of describing the extreme complexity of how our brain, body, and environment create perception.

Our eyes are not little HD (high-definition) cameras; our ears are not microphones. The way our brain filters sensual information is instead largely via prediction. When we see or hear anything at all, our brain shapes this information in light of everything we have previously experienced. It's only quite recently that we have discovered this about our sense perception—that it relies on what is called predictive processing, which I mentioned earlier. The dramatic implications of this discovery have yet to be absorbed into popular consciousness.

Crucially, our autonomic nervous system changes how these filters shape our perception. When we are stressed, our perception changes to highlight threat and danger. When we are relaxed and socially engaged this opens the scope of our perception so that we are more receptive to nuance and the symbolic nature of the world. We literally see the world in a different way. Our perception of what we assume to be objective reality changes according to our internal state. When we feel safe and curious, we begin to notice the aliveness of the world around us. We can start to see beneath the surface of things, to sense the vividness of Indra's Net as it unfolds around us.

This can be described as shifting our perception from *seeing* to *beholding*. This change in perception presents a world to us beyond the immediate threat of survival. It brings us into closer intimacy

---

*The idea that mythical and symbolic ways of being and knowing have evolved over many generations of cultural change is supported by many evolutionary thinkers and scientists. For a clear exploration of this theme, see David Sloan Wilson, *This View of Life* (New York: Alfred A. Knopf, 2019). From this perspective, the richest reservoir of cultural wisdom lies in the oldest indigenous cultures, such as the Indigenous Australian people. The work of Tyson Yunkaporta exemplifies this.

with the world, precipitating a sense of belonging and being a part of something wondrous. Indeed, it's not only a sense of belonging that is felt but a conjoining as well; a clear-as-day participation with the coming into being of the world. Our perception unshackles itself from the clutch of being a survivor and connects with the unbridled creativity of the world.

This feeds a greater sense of wonder, joy, and appreciation for our lives. In turn, these feelings act as a type of resourcing, strengthening our resilience and buffering us from the sharp edge of life. Wonder bonds us to the world, it opens and connects us to other people. It creates what John Vervaeke calls a reciprocal opening.* As we open to the world around us, the world responds in kind. The bonding and opening to life are two-way; the world is savoring its fragrance through relationship.

This dialogue with life breaks the profound, existential loneliness that occurs when we get stuck in a survivalist state. The simple joy and appreciation of being alive and in a living relationship with the world communicates an equally profound sense of knowing—that everything is okay, that we are safe in this present moment.

This implicit message from nature can be thought of as ecological communitas. Being in commune and shared breath with the world gives sustenance to the socially isolated, such as the mountain hermit. It helps feed the need for social community, warding off loneliness and despair. This is a key feature of the Golden Elixir practice, which allows people to remain sane and social through long periods of isolation.

The ability to drop into a deep sense of safety and rest is also a

---

*This term was coined by Vervaeke in response to Marc Lewis's model of reciprocal narrowing, which he describes as a key mechanism in addiction. As the work of Gabor Maté clearly demonstrates, there is a strong overlap between addiction and trauma. Reciprocal opening parallels the idea that "the opposite of addiction is not sobriety . . . the opposite of addiction is connection," given by Johan Hari—whereas interpersonal connection is essential for healing, 4E Cognitive Science would posit that reforging connection and belonging with our world around us is also key.

primary aspect of self-healing. This is one of the reasons why sleep is so important for our health and well-being. However, there are many social and cultural habits that are also vitally important for our health and for maintaining a sense of reciprocity, friendship, and play within our lives.

For instance, simple chatting and joking, laughing and merrymaking, are potently therapeutic and enrich our lives in ways that can't be measured. Everyday social activities like sports, exercise, bathing and sauna, cooking and dining, music, dance, ritual, and prayer—these all fulfill our lives and also keep our nervous system in states that are healing and regenerative. All these relational activities cue our nervous systems away from feeling like we're in a fight for survival. As the saying goes, when we can switch from survival to revival, we lay the groundwork for deep healing.

This is also the first step in many traditions of meditation and contemplative practice—to come to a state of deep rest so that we might revive ourselves. And in both the ancient Indic and Chinese traditions, self-massage was used to help bring us into this state of relaxation, safety, and contentment. Dien Chan can therefore shift our mode of being toward healing and also open our senses so we can greater savor and delight in the simple pleasures of life.

When we practice self-massage, we're soothing ourselves and cueing our bodies into the healing mode. With Dien Chan, we are specifically releasing the tension surrounding our eyes, ears, nose, and mouth. As we practice, we can also mindfully bring our senses into retreat, which can deactivate the habit of unconsciously scanning our environment for threat. This can also create a pattern interrupt from addictive technology and the need to always have sensual stimulation, meaning that if we find ourselves incessantly checking our emails or phones, we can use Dien Chan to restore our attention and calm our hearts. More broadly, it helps deactivate the yearning for greater and greater dopamine hits that underlie many addictive spirals. Instead of setting up a situation where we need more and more pleasure to experience joy, we reverse this dynamic so we can experience more and more joy in our simple, everyday lives.

The Dien Chan meditations for sensory retreat from the previous chapter help to quiet and soften the glare of our overly stimulated nervous systems. With practice, this can gradually reset our perception. The greater we can drop into a state of calm and equanimity, the more this temporary fasting of our vision and hearing can be thought of as cleaning, purifying, and refreshing the senses. Returning to the world out there can create the impression of perceiving with more clarity. When we can look at life with fresh eyes, we're less susceptible to old patterns of attention and more energized toward the invisible.

This is where things get interesting, for not only do we increase our mindfulness of the world, but so long as we can maintain a state of relative relaxation and safety, we can also enter into new ways of engaging and participating with the world around us. The move from a superficial seeing to a mythical beholding entails a voyage into the non-ordinary. This way of silver branch beholding holds considerable resonance with many other spiritual traditions.

Instead of seeing only the surface of things, we behold the subtle resonance that connects everything around us. But, if we limit ourselves to what is only superficially apparent, the richness and potentiality of life tends to get flattened, and we end up blinding ourselves to what's really before us. Forests are reduced to mere acres of timber, animals to kilos of meat, and other people to human resources.

The quantification of life reduces everything into familiar boxes, which has utilitarian value. But it also cuts out all the unknown unknowns, the bewildering possibilities of life. If we can create a reciprocal opening in our perception, we can stay attuned to the greater meaning and potential in life. We can reach a transjective stance, one that stays true to both the objective quantities and subjective qualities of life.

This is not simply a poetic way of being in the world. It's also more advantageous to our growth and survival as people, for it enables us to forge stronger kinships within our social circles. The heart and value of friendship isn't purely in one another's utility to each other. Evolution and a spiritual vision of life need not be alien to each other.

Like the mythical symbol of Indra's Net, the silver branch is an image from ancient Irish mythology. It comes from the story known as "The Voyage of Bran," first recorded in the eighth century. The telling recounts a wondrous music that suddenly appears to Bran but is always heard elusively at his back. He then discovers its source: a silver branch, adorned with clear, white blossoms. It's suggested that the music of the silver branch is what the great hero of Irish myth, Finn MacCool, called the music of what is.

Again, this speaks to a threshold being passed from seeing to beholding, from hearing to listening. The effect of this music precipitates a wild sequence of events, taking Bran to encounter the high seas, the son of the God of the Sea, Manannan Mac Lir. Whereas normal people see the ocean as a vast, gray, dangerous body of water, Manannan Mac Lir sees the ocean as a Plain of Delights.

Where normal perception entails a closing in on the known, silver branch perception evokes awe, wonder, and delight—an opening to all that is invisible around us and within us, an illuminated sensitivity and receptivity to the world. This change in perception is associated with the ancient Irish notion of *imbas,* the wisdom that is born from hearing, "the music of what is." This resonates strongly with the Huayan description of the Ocean Seal Samadhi—the whole world as a marvelous display of jewel-like, ever-blossoming inter-being. This is actually the only description we have of the way the Buddha perceived the world in the immediate aftermath of his enlightenment—as a perfect reflection of oceanic vastness and inter-being. Moriarty even makes an oblique reference to this by saying that "it is because of the clutching hawk talons in our hands that we cannot bring the world-mirroring water to our mouths."[2]

It also has a resonance with Daoist Golden Elixir practices, wherein there is the common goal of transmuting our immediate experience so that we're able to behold the full splendor of the world. Like myth in general, this process is occurring on many levels. It's something we can catch an inkling of by engaging with what brings us reverie, absorption, and wonderment. This is what the Dien Chan meditations later in this chapter can help make available to us.

On another level, the full absorption states that occur at the extreme depths of rapture and reverie are also known to awaken what is called extrasensory perception, such as precognition, remote viewing, clairvoyance, and clairaudience.

In traditional language these are called Siddhis; the spiritual powers that are born from deep practice. The clarity and luminosity of the sense bases, which increase through these hermetic endeavors, do indeed open the world in strange and unusual ways. Rather than dismiss the outer reaches of our sensory powers, I believe that we must heed the people who report back to us from visionary and ecstatic experience. After all, mystical experience is not rare in humans but is instead remarkably common. There's a social taboo against what lies beyond conventional understanding.

Typically, a degree of caution is recommended when engaging with these types of practice, because a common effect is for the practices to quickly go to one's head. The yearning for Siddhi and superpowers is very common in the yogic and qigong worlds. The Daoist countermeasure is to safeguard one's spirit within the Dan Tien—within the abdomen and center of the body.

This downward flow, which grounds us in equanimity, ensures we don't get ahead of ourselves. I wholeheartedly recommend people to be open to the possibility that the world is a Plain of Delights and not simply what we assume it to be. The alchemy of perception that's available to us is not only natural and transformative, but I strongly suspect it plays a key role in our future evolution as well.

◆ ◆ ◆

Our everyday perception is framed by its human limitations, in that we have only a certain amount of sense receptors, taste buds, and optical cones. This perceptual scope is termed the *human umphelt* and is quite distinct from how a dog or a snake perceives the world. However, just like we have the ability to increase our vagal tone and interact with our autonomic nervous system as it cascades into our perception, we also have the ability to widen our personal umphelt.

This process of noticing more detail and becoming aware of the aesthetic richness in our surroundings is similar to what Barrett calls emotional granularity. We move from a relatively pixilated view of the world to a high-definition experience. Or, conversely, the world transforms from a place of mechanical pixilation to a field of resonant vibration. This opening of the umphelt depends on our ability to be curious and in awe, which in turns rests on a foundation of feeling safe in our nervous system and mind-body. But, when we are in a fight for survival, the beautiful and majestic become irrelevant, as if drained from the world.

If we are continually in a state of survival, this influences both our ability to enjoy and savor life, as well as skews the way we interpret the meaning of our human stories. There's a slide into nihilism, cynicism, and apathy—a reciprocal closing that's associated with addiction and depression. An important example of this is recorded by Charles Darwin himself, who experienced a profound aesthetic disenchantment in his later years.

I have said that in one respect my mind has changed during the last twenty or thirty years. Up to the age of thirty, or beyond it, poetry of many kinds, such as the work of Milton, Gary, Byron, Wordsworth, Coleridge, and Shelley, gave me great pleasure, and even as a schoolboy I took intense delight in Shakespeare, especially in the historical plays. I have also said that formerly pictures gave me considerable, and music very great delight. But for many years I cannot endure to read a line of poetry: I have tried lately to read Shakespeare and found it so intolerably dull that it nauseates me. I have also lost my taste for pictures or music. . . . My mind seems to have become a kind of machine for grinding general laws out of large collections of facts, but why this should have caused the atrophy of that part of the brain alone, on which the higher tastes depend, I cannot conceive. . . . The loss of these tastes is a loss of happiness, and may possibly be injurious to the intellect, and more probably to the moral character, by enfeebling the emotional part of our nature.[3]

It's interesting that Darwin associated this aesthetic atrophy with our emotional nature. It's as if the "survival of the fittest" paradigm had become so entrenched in his nervous system that his entire sensitivity to the world had been rewired to perceive only the cold facts. But, the cold facts do not reflect the deep truth.

Data is meaningless without interpretation. And, interpretation is inseparable from imagination. This is one of the reasons why Corbin's notion of the imaginal is so useful, for it gives us a way to frame the interaction that happens between the world, our perception, and the imagination. In other words, all the predictive and intuitive functions of our brain and body emerge only through participation and interaction with the world. Ironically, instead of interpreting life only through a lens of survival, our actual survival depends on drawing from our full, imaginative capabilities. This means beauty and music are nontrivial—they support healing and growth both personally and collectively.

Iain McGilchrist's thesis states that the cultural dominance of the left hemisphere's way of perceiving the world has skewed our collective meaning-making, resulting in the many crises of the modern age. Our collective trauma has placed us firmly in a stance of survival, which means that we blind ourselves to the greater meaning, truth, and significance the world continually presents us with. We tend to interpret life, both in our literal sensory perception and our overarching meaning-making, through a lens of threat detection. It's not just our ways of thinking and speaking that reinforce a scarcity and survival mind-set, but our nervous system and embodiment equally color our world in this way.

We must reclaim a more balanced way of framing ourselves, both individually and culturally, within our stories. I describe this as a remembrance of our original face. The left hemisphere, and the very real drive for survival, are, of course, vital to our lives. But the right hemisphere, which opens us to our full embodiment, also opens us to possibility, risk, adaptation, and aesthetic arrest. It allows us to be captured by the wonder of the world.

We have the power to change how we see, both literally and mythopoetically. This endeavor isn't undertaken by simply paying attention to the surface of things. The attitude to aesthetics must shift from the default statement of "entertain me." There's an active participation that takes us beyond passive observation, or as Martin Shaw says, "Curiosity is a discipline of labor." With repetition and patience, the feeling of curiosity transforms into awe, reverie, and wonder. Repetition familiarizes what is alien, difficult, and uncomfortable.

A golden key to opening ourselves to this kind of captivation involves an embodied sense of connection through our heart. It doesn't occur by fixating on our sense organs or surface perception. This key is revealed if we look at the Chinese character for *listening,* which is composed of both the characters for *ear* and *heart.*

Keeping connected to the heart means that we continuously activate the downward flow, maintaining both a grounded embodiment and a calm and equanimous presence. This opens the senses to the peripherals—to all that is at the edge of our perception. It shifts us away from the laser-focused particularity of detecting threat and toward the embrace of our relational nature. Being embodied from the heart opens us to feeling embedded in the aesthetic richness of the world.

Khalil Gibran felt this when he wrote, "Beauty is not in the face, beauty is a light in the heart." In both Buddhist and Daoist understanding there is a subtle anatomy that lies behind the more physical structures of our sense organs and nerves. This anatomy won't be discovered through dissection but can be felt through direct experience.

At the finest level of consciousness there lies what are termed the *sense bases*, which are experienced in meditation as a luminosity directly behind each sense organ. If our awareness is sensitive enough, we can feel these just behind the eyes, ears, nose, and mouth. However, the master sense base does not rest in the head but rather in the space of the heart organ. Specifically, the heart base, termed the *hadaya vathu* in Pali scripture, resides in the lower chambers of the heart.

The downward flow allows us to drop into this space and I believe has a crude parallel with what we call vagal tone and heart rate variability. The quality of both our consciousness and our perception is determined when the state of our heart base is calm, still, and quiet. It sets the background tone for how our nervous system participates with the world.

The essence of a great many spiritual traditions lies in letting go of any heaviness and clenching from the heart base. The more we can relax the chest, the easier our breath becomes. The more we can empty the heart and become like clear vessels to our experience, the more our perception of self and world changes. This can create a fundamental shift toward feeling safe in our bodies, and in the world around us, which is the key to activating our innate self-healing and regenerative power.

However, the more we open to this process, the more the world opens to us. It's as if we enter into a more direct experience of the world that has less separation between subject and object, between me and other. As our perception becomes more interlinked with the coming into being of the world around us, we feel an increasing sense of connection. We feel embedded in the whole, and this gifts us with a sense of being at home wherever we are, of feeling an innate belonging to our lives.

The social dimension to this is called inter-being or, in more modern language, interpersonal neurobiology. We coexist with those around us in more enmeshed ways than we might assume. And the degree to which our individuality feels enmeshed with the world changes according to our embodiment: when we observe from the head, we feel separate and disconnected; when our perspective is also rooted in the heart and belly, we come into participation, connection, and reciprocity.

Although this way of understanding our perception and consciousness is only beginning to be mapped out in the outlier branches of cognitive science and things like polyvagal theory, indigenous wisdom traditions offer us a wealth of knowledge from generations of accumulated direct experience.

In qigong and the Golden Elixir practice, what I have termed the *downward flow* is essentially our ability to connect to the Earth. This is closely related to our physical balance—what is called rooting or *song* in traditional qigong—and reflects our ability to come to rest and feel deeply relaxed. This is our yin energy—our ability to remain calm and grounded. The more we can relax our body, the more the Earth responds back, rising to support us.

This feeling of the Earth as a vast presence underneath us is often described as a type of mother energy, an archetypal emanation of unconditional love and acceptance, that is at once very real but at the same time beyond normal modes of comprehension. It cuts through all the tragedy in our lives and somehow gifts us with a sense that everything is okay, despite the raging storms of the world around us. Shifting into a silver branch mode of perception allows us to listen deeply and develop a relationship with the Earth. (Please see appendix C see for a fuller exploration of the many faces of the Earth.)

There's also an upward current of energy that connects us in new ways to everything above us. The natural response when we look up to a sky full of stars, or to the dazzling light of the sun and moon, is that of wonder and awe. This is our yang energy—our ability to be open to possibility and inspiration—our ability to jump up and rise to each occasion. Whereas the downward flow is associated with the out-breath and a resting back into the vagus, our yang energy keeps us upright and draws fresh in-breaths, connecting us to all the inspiration and wonder in the world.

Our yang energy lights up consciousness and illuminates our sense bases. It allows us to take in the newness of the world and therefore is vital to discovering new ways of seeing and for shifting from curiosity to wonder and delight.

In qigong, this ability to connect to wonder and welcome in fresh energy is embodied through the crown of our heads. This is why the classic postural instruction is to imagine your head being suspended from a golden thread, which creates a sense of naturally lifting and aligning the spine. When all the physical and energetic pathways to the head are open and flowing, we are allowed a greater receptivity to the world around us. This is why the term for lifting from the head is sometimes called Ting Jin, or listening energy, as if the crown of the head is light, spacious, and open to the sky.

This quality is supported through the expression of our face and head, both physically and in our awareness. If our head is aligned upon the spine with as little unnecessary force and tension as possible, this helps increase circulation, flow, and receptivity. Self-massage is one way to help achieve this, but postural exercises are also very helpful.

For our face, there is another key postural instruction: place the tip of the tongue on the roof of the mouth, just behind the front teeth. This frames the mouth and the jaw so we can relax without losing the face's natural poise. It keeps a sense of buoyancy through our centerline. It also encourages correct breathing (through the nose) and stimulates the salivary glands.

Our yang energy naturally flows toward the head, and when it's not grounded in the body, all sorts of imbalances, like emotional agitation, anxiety, insomnia, and headaches can be created. For this reason, the primary step in qigong, and also in the pathway to healing, is to ground our energy and come into a sense of relaxation and safety.

Once we've established this switching of the nervous system, we can perceive our bodies and lives with more clarity. This sense of clarity is called the clear yang and is fundamental to adapting and changing with the world around us. It echoes what many philosophers have mused, that evil behavior is primarily a matter of ignorance; therefore, clarity of perception is essential for goodness and social harmony. It also keeps our spine from slouching in with the downward flow, as it lifts us and keeps us awake. For if we really were to totally relax our face and body, our mouth would go slack jawed, our head would drop forward, and our body would tumble to the ground. We would essentially fall asleep and lose consciousness.

So, there is a balance to be struck between the letting go and the welcoming in, between the downward and the upward vectors of our embodiment. The balancing of this natural poise acts as a bridge between the head and heart, between the major yin and yang channels of the body, and between the different layers of our nervous system. It also balances us between the existential undercurrents of safety and wonder.

If we view our nervous system and perception in a more global sense, we can think of the top of our head and the bottom of our pelvis as two poles that connect us to and resonate with the experiences of safety and wonder. The ground below us offers safety; the sky above us offers wonder. Maintaining an openness and balance through our whole centerline brings a sense of integration and coherence to our personhood.

In turn, this can initiate a process of unfolding from a stable sense of safety toward an all-encompassing, unconditional love, gratitude, and acceptance, naturally shifting us from embodiment to embeddedment. The courage to open ourselves and be curious precipitates greater and more expansive experiences of awe, wonder, delight, and reverie. Discovering our original face is becoming fully transparent to who we are—an ongoing process that transmutes the ordinary and commonplace into icons and symbols of the extraordinary.

The following Dien Chan practices can be thought of as stepping-stones toward silver branch perception. We can use them to reconnect to the ever new—the aspects of ourselves that are yet to emerge—changing our perception so that we can savor the simplicity and sensuality of the world with greater appreciation and delight. It can also therapeutically prompt us toward more joyful and kinder ways of behaving. When we come back to our senses, we have the opportunity to change how we see other people, learning to see further into the inter-being of collective trauma.

We can practice these techniques in a relatively short amount of time, and they can be a very helpful tool for clearing the charge that surrounds our heart and sense portals. But, if we bring these techniques into a meditation or contemplative practice, they can form the basis of great transformation. This is because the root of our negative emotional patterns resides at the sense bases and alight each time our perception touches something that resonates with these old patterns. This is why equanimity is the greatest key to unlocking the stories that confine us. Equanimity reconfigures our perception toward a more truthful beholding of the world.

Whereas some people might assume that perceiving everything through a lens of equanimity would nullify our enjoyment of life—would make everything gray and bland—actually the opposite is true. Equanimity opens us to wonder. It does not mute the flavors of life but rather is a conductor of bliss. It's a stripping away of all lenses and false artifice.

The natural responses to a world in full disclosure are love, appreciative joy, compassion, and wonder. This is our default mode once our survivalist mentality is switched off, once our appetites are temporarily satiated. We enter a world of reciprocity, of creative participation and collaboration, rather than one of pure rivalry and competition. This shift in perception opens us to vistas that are much wider and grander than the scope of analytic or anatomical thinking. The symbol of the face is made translucent, or, as Rumi says, "We are the mirror as well as the face in it."

DIEN CHAN MEDITATIONS
FOR CURIOSITY, WONDER, AND DELIGHT

🌸 Opening Eyes of Fire

1. Rub the palms until there is a noticeable warmth and charge in the hands.

2. Place the palms over the eyes, resting the eyelids, and relaxing the eyes.

3. Use the tips of the index fingers to press on the point BL1/*Jing Ming*/ Bright Eyes, circling each way two to three times (see figure 11.2, step 1, on page 165).

4. Stimulate all the points around the eye's orbit, creating a figure-eight pattern. Reverse.

5. Stimulate the points BL2/*Zhan Zhu*/Gathered Bamboo, *Yu Yao*/ Fish Loin, TB23/*Si Zhu Kong*/Silken Bamboo Hollow, GB1/*Tong Zi Liao*/Bone of New Vision, and ST1/*Cheng Qi*/Receiving Tears (see figure16.1).

6. Use the pads of the index fingers to sweep above and beneath the eyes, clearing away any stagnation and sediment.

7. Use the pads of the fingers to sweep down either side of the nose and away across the cheeks.

8. Repeat steps 1 and 2. While the palms rest over the eyes, with the eyes closed, turn your eyes to look left, right, up, down, and at each corner.

9. While the palms are completely covering the ocular orbit, so it's as dark as possible, open the eyes and look toward every direction in turn. Imagine that any heat from the eyes is releasing outward.

10. Keeping the eyes closed, use the palms and fingers to sweep away any tension from the eyes and wash downward across the face and neck. Then, as slowly as possible, open your eyes, paying attention to both your vision and how the eyes feel.

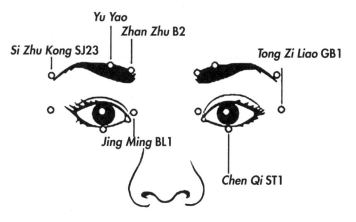

Figure 16.1. Eyes of Fire—points to increase circulation and open the energetics around the eyes

The Dien Chan Meditations for Curiosity, Wonder, and Delight exercise has multiple functions. Its roots come from the Chinese massage therapy techniques that were instigated nationally in China through the 1970s to improve eyesight and prevent macular degeneration. Not only does it help increase circulation to the eyes, but it also helps improve clarity of vision. Aesthetically, this is a great exercise to clear any puffiness or bags under the eyes, refreshing tired or sore eyes.

Energetically, we are opening all the channels that start and finish around the eyes, and so this exercise helps boost circulation to Bladder, Stomach, Gall Bladder, and San Jiao acupuncture channels. Holographically, the area around the eye has particular resonance with the reproductive organs and so is especially helpful in working with any gynecological issue. It also has resonance with the heart and lungs and so can help optimize breathing, lung health, and heart function.

The eyes, unlike the other sensory organs, form an extension of the brain. The creation of our vision constitutes up to 30 percent of all brain function. This places the eyes in a slightly separate category from our other sensory organs. In traditional qigong theory, the eyes are unusual as they can be classified as pure yang, whereas the rest of the body can be classified as yin. This suggests that the eyes and our capacity for vision somehow carry the spark of life in a more vivid and powerful way. Indeed, qigong healers see the eyes as both passive receptors of the world, and active creators. Our vision can participate with life and transmit information to the world around us.

Neuroscience tells us that much of our vision is entirely simulated from the predictions made by our brains. This allows us to create a seamless image of the world, which would pass us by if we only relied on the technical capacity of our eyes. Rather than being able to detect the speed of a tennis ball, our eyes and brain predict its passage so that we can react with enough speed. Also, much of our peripheral vision and habitual environment relies on this predictive power, in large part because it reduces the amount of calories and energy needed for our brain to continuously create this high-definition world we see around us. This is perhaps one aspect of the active creation of the eyes that qigong masters refer to. They would take it one step further and suggest that consciousness is lighting up the world, and by increasing our conscious awareness of the world, we can also light up the world in unique ways.

This is what is sometimes called awakening eyes of fire, for the intensity and life force of our gaze can be a powerful attribute in both our social life and in how we envision the world around us. Aesthetically, the mythic complexity, relational beauty, and symbolic depth of the world can be activated by changing the way we see. The Opening Eyes of Fire exercise can help open this capacity.

🌿 Opening Ears of Water

1. Rub the palms until there is a noticeable warmth and charge in the hands.

2. Swiftly rub the ears with the palms for ten to twenty seconds.

3. Use the thumb and forefinger to pinch and curl out the outer ear, from the top to the bottom, pulling the ear lobes downward. Repeat three times.

4. Use the pad of the index or middle fingers to seal the ear hole, then press down and spiral outward from the inside to outside. Repeat three times.

5. Use the pad of the index or middle fingers to press upward behind the ear, from the bottom to the top. Repeat three times. Then press downward behind the ear. Repeat three times. Also repeat at the front of the ears.

6. Use the pads of both index and middle fingers to circle in the space underneath the ear and behind the jaw, softening and opening the circulation downward from the ear.

7. Bring awareness to your hearing and how your ears feel.

Performing the Opening Ears of Water exercise usually makes the ears feel very warm; the increase in blood circulation also boosts the circulation to the head. This is partly why stimulating points on the ears can positively affect and regulate blood pressure. In Chinese medicine, the ears are mirrors of the kidneys. Although this sounds unusual, the ears and kidneys develop from the same tissue source in utero. Not only do they share a similarity in shape, but they are embryologically twinned as well. It is for this reason that points on and around the ear have particular effect on the kidney energy, which in Chinese medicine is linked to our adrenal glands and is seen as the primary root of our energy. Massaging the ears acts as an energy booster and stress reducer.

The vagus nerve is also most superficially accessible within and just below the ear. It's for this reason that vagus nerve stimulation, which gives an electrical charge to this nerve, is implanted behind the earlobe. We can give more gentle stimulation to the vagus nerve through massaging the ears, and so this technique has many positive knock-on effects.

🪷 Three Breaths at the Threshold

1. Draw all your senses inward, resting your awareness at the bases of the sense organs, just behind the eyes, ears, nose, and heart. Keep your senses entirely receptive; do not extend outward, but keep your awareness attuned to the actual process of listening, seeing, smelling, and feeling.

2. Cup the palms over the eyes so that no light is observable. While your hands are still in place, open the eyes and make full 360-degree circles in both directions, as if releasing any heat from the eyes. Close the eyes and press the palms into the eyeballs, slowly sweeping outward over the temples. (It's helpful to slightly raise the eyebrows to create a nice seal between the hands and ocular ridge.)

3. Keeping the eyes closed, gently pat the palms over the eyes for the count of three slow breaths. (Do not pat the actual eyeball; rather, cup the hands, and pat the palms on the upper and lower ridges around the eyes.) Release the palms and very gently open the eyes and keep your attention entirely rested on the sense bases, unblinking, for three breaths. Then relax your attention, gently blink, and notice any subtle change created in your way of seeing.

4. Cup the palms over the ears, blocking out external sound.

5. Rub the palms over the ears in circles and then quickly open the palms outward, as if unplugging the ears.

6. Gently pat the palms over the ears for a count of three slow breaths. Release the palms and keep your attention entirely on the sense bases for three breaths. Then relax your attention and notice any change in your hearing.

The Three Breaths at the Threshold exercise is used to refine our clarity of perception, to cleanse the windows of perception as it were. The clearer our state of awareness is while performing this exercise, the more effect it will create. Although we're honing all our attention within the ears and eyes, after this exercise we should pay special attention to bringing our awareness back into the trunk of the body—to ground ourselves.

Monkey Hands Enliven the Blood

1. Bring your left hand close to your left ear, placing the finger pads of your right hand upon the left palm. Shift your eyes to look toward your right periphery.
2. As you gaze to the right, rub your fingers up and down the palm, both listening with the left and gazing to the right. Switch hands to the other ear, gazing toward the left, and repeat. Go back and forth between each direction three to nine times on each ear.

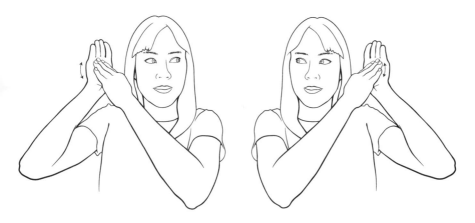

Figure 16.2. Monkey Hands Enliven the Blood

This technique is adapted from a Golden Elixir practice associated with Xing Yi Chuan, an internal martial art. By bringing a more direct attention into our sensory field outside the body, we begin to bridge the inner and outer. The movement of our eyesight into the periphery has a specific effect of opening toward wholeness and shifting out of the tunnel vision that is so typical of patterns of stress and fundamentalism.

This is something that has been discovered in EMDR therapy, which shows how changing our visual field while talking through stressful memories can reprogram our brain so that we are less entrapped in fixed patterns of thinking. In particular, horizontal eye movements have been researched to have the most powerful effect, harkening back to the origins of EMDR, which stemmed from taking walks in nature alongside therapy sessions.

When we are out in nature, our horizontal visual field is opened widely. This shifting between right and left might well have a balancing effect on the two hemispheres of the brain, which could explain why going for walks or running can have a clarifying effect on one's thoughts.

There's another facet to this exercise in that it bridges vision and hearing. Just like peripheral sight opens us toward wholeness, our hearing is linked to our nervous system. The high-frequency sound created through the rubbing of our palms also helps shift the nervous system out of fight-or-flight and toward the social engagement mode.

This has been documented by Stephen Porges's Safe and Sound program, which applies polyvagal theory in a therapeutic setting to shift autistic children into more socially open states. When we're stuck in a sympathetic dominant state, our nervous system is primed for threat detection, and this slackens our eardrums to become more alert to low-frequency sounds, like the rumbling growl of a tiger.

By attuning our ears to sonorous high-frequency sound, we help shift our nervous system into more healing and socially oriented states. When our eardrums tighten, we're able to hear human voices with more clarity, thereby improving our ability to discern tone, nuance, and intention in others' voices.

This points toward another method for using our senses to ground our nervous systems and calm our mind—music, and in particular, music that contains sonorous melody and singing.

❀ Embedded Listening

1. Close the eyes. Gently place your awareness simultaneously on each sense base and slowly draw your awareness from the eyes, ears, nose, and mouth inward to the center of the head.

2. Feel how being centered within your head can open the central axis of your body, feeling connected to the center of the heart and belly. Allow your awareness to rest and fill this central channel, from the base of your pelvis to the apex of your head (being equally aware of the two polarity points of our Mundus Axis—Ren1/*Hui Yin*/Seabed and Du20/*Bai Hui*/Hundred Meetings).

3. Gradually change these two points on the body so they are listening outward. Be receptive to everything above your head through your apex point. Be receptive to everything below your body through your base point.

4. As your finish this short exploration, see if you can retain this sense of two-way listening—open equally to inside-outside and above-below. Notice if this creates any change in how your body feels or the state of your mind.

The Embedded Listening exercise does not use massage but can be accessed with more ease by working with the other Dien Chan self-care techniques and meditations already introduced. Although it is a personal relationship that one has with the Earth beneath one's feet, my own experience suggests that by increasing our ability to feel down into the Earth, we can initiate a more harmonious relationship.

My tai chi teacher calls this making friends with gravity, and indeed the benefits for our general balance are great, especially going into old age where taking falls is a major health risk. However, once we've established that we do have a personal relationship with the Earth, and that

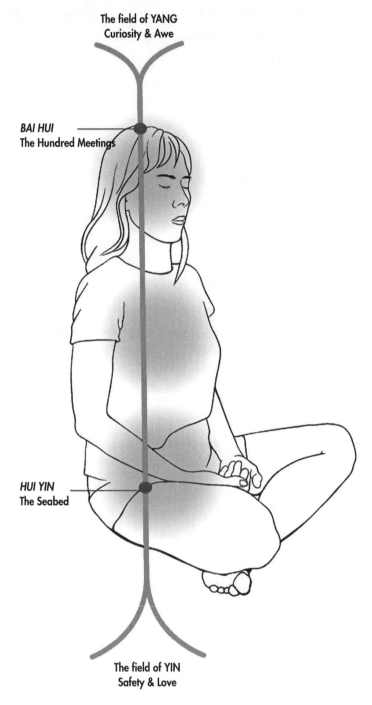

Figure 16.3. Embedded Listening

our lives very much depend on it, we are led into deeper and stranger relationships with what is beneath us.

The two primary ingredients in the sensorial alchemy of the Golden Elixir I have listed are safety and curiosity. There is, of course, great ambiguity in what these words actually mean for our inner lives. I would suggest that these two feelings can be extended and expanded outward, and that by shifting into an embedded listening, we can not only feel these ingredients inside of us but also as streaming into us from outside our bodies.

If we open to the Earth in such a way, it can rise up to support us. The safety of the Earth doesn't only support and steady our bodies, but it also nourishes and feeds us. As such, this feeling of safety can easily expand into a feeling of love. This is why all over the world the Earth is spoken of as a mother. If we listen deeply, there's a source of unconditional love that's always singing through us and uplifting us.

At the other end of the spectrum, if we open to the sky in such a way, it naturally strikes awe and wonder in us. The vastness of the sky is a natural source of wonder. Rilke echoes this in saying, "Illuminated in your infinite peace, a billion stars go spinning through the night, blazing high above your head." It's not simply our eyes that filter in this wonder, but our whole being is lit open to it—and the apex point of our body uniquely so.

In the same way that Dien Chan uses a natural resonance to mirror different parts of our body, we can harness this same resonance from within and harmonize with the fields of love and wonder in which we are embedded. My own experience suggests that not only is this happening regardless of what we think about emotion or consciousness, but that by giving the experience of love and wonder wide birth, this way of being in the world can be of great value both for our health and those around us.

❧ Tea Ceremony

1. Boil water.
2. Make tea.
3. Drink tea.

The difference between these simple steps, which most people are already very familiar with, and tea ceremony lies in the quality of our attention. Whereas most people make tea without really paying any attention to either step, if we increase our attention and mindfulness, we will notice that making and drinking tea offers us gifts for each sensory portal. More than this, the act of sharing tea has a unique ability to strengthen our connective capacity. Sharing a cup of tea, we can connect with others with greater ease.

If we are drinking living tea (high-quality loose-leaf tea), then we can find a connective bridge with nature. This is why tea has traditionally been so popular in Asian cities, for it can carry one back to the raw nature and fresh air of the mountains. Beyond this, if we approach tea as a ceremony or ritual, it is uniquely adapted to help connect us into a deeper relationship with our personhood, which is why tea and tea ceremony are so favored by Buddhists and Daoists.

Even though the culture that has evolved around tea ceremony has grown to include incredible nuance in how the water is treated, the equipment and handling of tea making, and the art of savoring tea, one can, in essence, use the above three steps as the primary instruction. Paying attention to each step, and not being distracted with anything else, can change the experience of drinking tea from consuming an everyday beverage to imbibing a sensory concerto.

If we listen with a degree of reverence to this concerto, the simple and mundane act of sipping tea can slowly reveal the extraordinary beauty of simply being in a human body. All our senses can play together, including listening to the sound of water, taking in the sight of fresh leaves and bright green liquor, and, of course, savoring the beautiful aromas and tastes.

Underneath these high notes of tea ceremony lie a deeper sensory melody, one that plays out through the textures and receptivity of our body. The interplay of external and internal sensation can be a vessel for the imagination, which can carry us into resonance with all the hidden dimensions of this simple tea leaf, connecting us to both forest and mountain.

These practices move sequentially from the more physical and body-bound to the more conscious and perceptual. We can use them in a simple and quick way if we need a light but immediate reset. Or we can go deeper and touch into the more subtle aspects of our perception. The right way is to go slowly and begin by spending only a brief amount of time on each practice. The greater our level of calmness and equanimity, the more we can sustain and lengthen the practice, which in turn will create more noticeable results. Whatever way we practice, there should always be an emphasis on finishing by grounding our awareness down through the body, as we don't want to accumulate any excess energy in the head. On the contrary, we aim to bring only the lightest and gentlest attention when working in these more subtle aspects of our mind-body.

The aim for these practices is not to produce some kind of psychedelic effect, to *see the light* as it were, but rather to bring the qualities of stillness, clarity, and spaciousness into our perception. To be clear-sighted about both the immediacy of our environment and the wider holistic context. There is a concurrence between our perception, state of mind, and physiology. When our social-orientation mode is grounded in safety but open to possibility, which means open to risk and vulnerability, we find ourselves more alive to the world and with more life energy coursing through our bodies. This can be powerfully therapeutic. It can also greatly enrich our lives, allowing us to savor, appreciate, and delight in both the ordinary and the extraordinary.

SEVENTEEN

. . . .

Bringing
It All Together

The origin is ever-present.

JEAN GEBSER

There are many ways to harness the power of the face; there are many ways to bring Dien Chan into your life. The sequences and techniques we have explored throughout this book offer a first stepping-stone toward your journey of discovering the original face. It is often said that the journey is more important than the destination, and in many ways the journey of developing our sensitivity, calmness, and curiosity are both the path and the reward. It's through this exploration that we will find the most accessible and relevant way to practice Dien Chan for ourselves, whether it's for de-stressing, healing, or self-realization.

Each person has a unique history and makeup, alongside different needs and goals. I hope you can find your own way to realize the potential of your own body and perception. In this regard, I offer some advice for how to best utilize Dien Chan and also how to adapt it to your day-to-day life.

1. DIEN CHAN AS A BRIDGE BETWEEN DIFFERENT MODES AND PHASES OF LIFE

Dien Chan can help us bridge between our different modes of being. The most apparent shift happens between our nighttime and daytime self. Dien Chan can help us wake up in the morning and can help clear and refresh our senses so that we can savor the day afresh. It can also be extremely helpful for bringing our bodies to rest and improving the quality of our sleep. This is especially so when practiced in tandem with good sleep hygiene, such as refraining from eating and bright light exposure a few hours before sleep.

If we are engaged in problem-solving or creative pursuits, Dien Chan can help us connect to our intuitive self, to spark curiosity and inspiration, and to think outside the box. It can switch us into our non-linear and polyrhythmic mode of being—what I have called our holographic self. This enables a playful listening, curiosity, and effortlessness in how we respond to the world.

It can also help switch on our socially engaged mode of being, where we are more attuned to other's faces, emotions, and intentions. I have called this the orientation toward beauty, where we seek mutual growth, integrity, and reciprocity in our relationships. Dien Chan can therefore be used in preparation for important or intimate meetings, or simply to calm ourselves and help us be present and openhearted in our relationships.

2. DIEN CHAN AS A DAILY PRACTICE

The beauty of Dien Chan is that it can be quick and easy to use. Therefore, it's simply a matter of remembrance and dedication to reap the benefits. Often this happens best by bringing it into existing routines. Dien Chan can easily be layered into washing and grooming or at the beginning or ending of other daily routines like meditation, yoga, or exercise.

We can choose to use Dien Chan spontaneously when we need, and this happens most easily when you have practiced and become familiar with the self-care exercises that resonate most with you. However, if we aim to use Dien Chan in a more methodical way—for healing or resetting our nervous system—for example, it cannot be overstated how important duration, repetition and patience are. To get the most powerful results from Dien Chan, we need to be consistent. A simple way to structure a consistent daily practice is to commit to twenty days in a row. Keeping a tally and can find the right pattern and rhythm, even if it's only for a few minutes a day, will accumulate a much stronger effect than if we only have one big session every now and then.

3. DIEN CHAN AS AN INSTIGATOR OF WONDER

We can use Dien Chan as a way to remind ourselves of the beauty and mystery of the world. That part of us that is completely natural and indigenous to the world can be reawakened and refreshed via Dien Chan. Like watering a seed, if we bring fresh water to our perception, we can discover new ways, new angles, and new perspectives in our lives. It's this continuous renewal and regeneration that keeps us growing, healing, and motivated by the future.

I would say that this ability to draw ourselves into wonder and to be drawn into awe is my favorite thing about Dien Chan. Instead of being consumed by the past or using Dien Chan only to avert catastrophe, we can practice Dien Chan out of sheer joy—just because it feels good, brings pleasure, and brightens the spirits. In turn, this spirit of enjoying life spreads through our perception, opening old songs, fragrances, and tastes to fresh delight and appreciation.

These three pointers are worth exploring individually but come into full potency when taken as one. The virtues of a daily practice, of being able to transition and flow and of being awake to wonder—these are all connected. For within each daily repetition, we seek to practice as if for the first time, with curiosity and sensitivity to the felt body. And to be fully open to the flow state, to the seamless spontaneity of life, we must be alert to the unknown wonders of the moment.

When we start to behold the whole world as an icon—that is, the mythic and symbolic dimensions of our everyday lives—we relate to other people in a way that honors our full relationality. This means we see others not only at face value but also with a more mature level of empathy, with an understanding and appreciation of the shared trouble, struggle, and trauma that all peoples bear somewhere inside of them.

Instead of seeing trauma as a misfortune that only the unlucky and downtrodden endure, we recognize that life is inherently traumatic, that death is an ever-present reality and force of transformation. In this sense, we are all the walking wounded. Coming in to a post-tragic way of being, so that we don't revert to a naive idealism or get stuck in a vicious circle, enables us to behold the world afresh and with appreciation. It also calls forth a type of radical compassion that gives strength and courage to reconcile and heal the war-torn parts of ourselves and our communities.

This is where Dien Chan opens new pathways in our relationships. Instead of mimicking the subtle expressions of fear, anxiety, disgust, and anger that we sometimes encounter in others' faces, we can choose to see into the transformative potential of others. This transformative potential is sometimes called the better angels of our nature.

We seek to see other people not at face value but to behold their angelic nature. Polyvagal theory speaks to this and highlights a kind of ordinary wisdom: the way we express ourselves to others can actively transform the other person. Wolfgang Goethe wonderfully describes this interpersonal alchemy. To paraphrase him, if we treat someone merely as they are or appear to be, they remain as they appear to be.

But, if we treat someone as they might be or ought to be, we help them reveal all their unknown potential.

Crucially, this doesn't mean that we project onto others our idealized version of what we would like to see in them. To demand high standards in other people's behavior is one thing, but to always expect perfect behavior is a setup for great disappointment. Rather, it means that we hold a kind of negative capability toward others, meaning we see each person as continuously on a threshold and that we can help each other grow into the unknown and unexpected. Each person has within them the potential for transformation. At the deep end, each person is always on the cusp of awakening to reservoirs of wonder, joy, and love that were in the previous moment entirely nonexistent. Our own openness to the unknown can guide others toward new and spontaneous experiences.

By reserving space for others to unshackle themselves from all the patterns of the past, we can then participate with and encourage a newness and sudden vitality in ourselves, others, and the world around us. This is where personal growth and healing occur—in the relationships between beings, not only within each individual.

This fluid dynamic between us and the world has been called the imaginal—it ties our emotional makeup into the workings and faces of others. It threads together the threshold that each face represents. It's in this sense that Corbin calls the imagination an organ of perception. It envisages both what is and what might be at the same time, an interaction that reflects our inter-being.

I believe this orientation brings us closer to our most angelic future versions of ourselves; it gives space for the Buddha-nature that arises in all beings. In more certain terms, it cultivates goodwill, friendship, and sustainable relationships. From this angle, this approach to ourselves, other people, and the world is both a feature of religion in its original essence and also of science as an aspirational process. The work of Pierre Teilhard de Chardin, and its updated evolutionary framework given by

David Sloan Wilson, show us that this silver branch perception isn't merely an artistic dream but also a global leap in planetary evolution. The grandeur of this statement can be brought home by the fact that we can participate in this leap with each face we encounter and in the most ordinary moments of our day.

When we speak of resonance and the imaginal, we may think this is happening behind the scenes, in some abstract dreamworld that underpins the solid material world. But, the imaginal is tethered to our biology. It's just as much an evolutionary process as it is a creative and poetic one. It is happening right now on our faces and upon the face of the world. Bringing this wonder into our everyday world is therefore a life-affirming and healing pursuit.

Dien Chan can help us remember this often forgotten brilliance in our lives. It offers a way of recalibrating our perception toward newness, regeneration, and joyful spontaneous creativity.

CONCLUSION

• •

An Orientation
toward Beauty

There are several different currents of thought tied together in this book. These currents come from very different worldviews, but hopefully the comparisons I have given show that a cohesion and harmony can be made from what might at first seem disparate. Beyond this, I hope that the actual self-care practices give a real embodied sense of how we can change both our physiology and spirit through our own agency. This is one of the key virtues of Dien Chan—that we can come in touch with our own self-healing power. We can assist and support not only the inherent wisdom in our biology, but we also can affirm a way of seeing and relating to the world that aspires to what is both individually healthy, socially harmonious, and in ecological kinship.

The reason I connect our personal health outward into the health of our family, society, and environment is because this expansion from embodiment to embeddedness is actually key to our self-healing power. There's a fractal pattern that moves outward from our face into the world, and at the same time inward into the inner worlds of our body. How can my personal health be separate from the health of the land or the vibrancy of the food and water I make a part of me?

Feeling our whole body together as one opens a spaciousness in our being, allowing us to release the particular points of contraction, whether it be blood flow stagnation or emotional fixity. Our boundedness within our bodies and our boundaries with the world become more porous and interdependent. Whole and part enter into a flow, and what was once fragmented becomes coherent and integrated. At the same time, this felt connection through our whole body connects and attunes us to the field of natural regeneration in which we are embedded. By connecting to nature, we connect to the body's inherent capacity for self-healing.

We can connect to nature both through listening more fully to our own bodies and by extending our senses and attention to the sounds, sights, aromas, tastes, and touch of the natural world around us. Birdsong, the sound of ocean waves, the aroma of woodlands after rainfall, the warmth of the sun—all these sensations carry nature's healing message of change and transformation. By listening with not just one sense, but with all our senses as a whole, we can tune our body toward this healing frequency.

It's my understanding that Dien Chan helps shift us toward wholeness, and this feeling of wholeness and connection attunes us to nature's regenerative impulse. In Vietnam, Dien Chan is primarily a form of therapy and self-healing, but my experience of framing Dien Chan within the greater meditative and qigong traditions shows that Dien Chan can also be a helpful tool in cultivating a more open, truthful, and wise perception of reality. And so the journey of healing stress and rewriting emotional patterns crosses over into a journey of renewing our sense of delight in the ordinary beauty of life.

Being content and at peace with how things are and appear to be paradoxically gives space for the creative blossoming of life's potential. By not interfering with the world or willing it to be different we actually initiate a process of growth and evolution. This does not mean that we're completely detached or indifferent but rather that we are open to all that's unknown in our shared future. It's for this reason that the wisdom teachings, which prescribe a level of equanimity and detachment, are said to have a medicinal effect on our lives. Changing our self-perception and our relationships affects our biology in significant ways.

However, it's often the case that we cannot overcome illness or trauma entirely by ourselves. It takes a team effort and wisdom to be able to discern to what extent self-healing is accessible. Our environment plays an important role in this accessibility, for if we are cut off from a natural environment, it becomes increasingly difficult to remember what spring, autumn, sunrise, and a night full of stars really feels like in our mind-body. Nature-deficit syndrome is not to be underestimated. Likewise, without the touch of friendship and family, we might forget how we came to be in this world, as communal creatures.

Changing the way we see ourselves and the way we talk and react to other people is no mean feat. As such, I would like to reiterate that Dien Chan is most helpful when framed within an ecology of practices and healing modalities. Although Dien Chan does have potency all by itself, a truly holistic approach to health includes our diet (nutritional, informational, and technological), exercise and sleep, social nourishment, and connection to nature. The beauty of Dien Chan is that it can fuse into many different practices and aspects of our lives. By working directly with our senses we both reconfigure our perception of the world and in turn change how the world sees our own face.

In the Mayan Tzutujil language, the word for *face* is the same word used for *fruit*. There's a layered understanding that the fruit we bear to the world is possible only through a familial connection with the world. Our faces stem from many generations of ancestral growth, and intertwined in this fruition is a secret ingredient, one of unbridled creativity and wonder. This willingness to face the world with a sense of unique possibility, awe, and wonder is what carries us out from the shadow of our genetic heritage and into the unknown. Not only do we contain the seed for the next hundred thousand generations, but we also bring fresh water to its fruition with how we choose to express and look upon one another.

This marks the tricky balance of equanimity that we bring to life's pleasures and pains. If we go off the deep end and become recluses amid others, we risk turning our equanimity into something else, something that is more akin to nihilism and apathy. But, if we find the right balance of equanimity in our everyday relationships, we can actually come to savor all the simple things in life with relish and joy. We can come to savor the deliciousness of the world without becoming embroiled in or fueling the trouble that can so often ensue. This ability to savor life opens a natural source of wonder in us, and it's this sense of wonder that makes way for new life, healing, and regeneration.

APPENDIX A

· ·

On Tools &
Point Stimulation

The use of massage tools in Dien Chan is one of the key characteristics of how it's practiced in Vietnam. However, I have chosen to emphasize the empty-handed techniques in this book to make Dien Chan as easy and accessible as possible. We can achieve great results simply using our hands, fingertips, and knuckles. It's not necessary to have any special tools, especially if they are difficult to obtain. However, there are also certain limitations to empty-handed techniques; we can't create the same pinpoint pressure that a small tool can achieve. In Vietnam, Professor Bui Quoc Chau has invented a wide range of tools that are designed to create unique effects that would be challenging or impossible to create with only our hands. The use of moxibustion, vibratory tools, electronic tools, and even ice tools are clear examples. There are also hammer/percussive tools, Gua Sha tools, rake tools, cooling rollers, spiky rollers, tools for different parts of the body—it is a veritable feast of invention and innovation.

Out of the wide range of tools available, the primary and original tool that is most important for treatment is the simple point probe. This is used to stimulate the points of the face. It's used in the same way that a fingertip would be used to press on a point; however, its surface area is much smaller than a fingertip, and so a greater force can be projected into the point. Because of this, it becomes easier to identify what may be called the living point, or ah-shi point. These points of heightened sensitivity create stronger responses through the mind-body. This type of tool is relatively easy to find if you search the internet for a "massage point probe." It's also very easy to improvise and use any object that has a smoothly tipped edge or point. At the very extreme would be a toothpick or acupuncture needle, which are obviously too sharp, and so, ideally, we are looking for a point surface of two to five millimeters. A small, smooth stone, chopstick, or the smooth end of a pen are very accessible substitutes.

The way to use a point stimulator is similar to how you would use a fingertip to press on a point. Because there are some excellent books and apps (refer to the ones mentioned in the Using This Book section, see page 13) already available that go into great detail about specific point prescriptions, I will only describe the way to use this tool. Once we have a feel for it, we can discover point combinations that are uniquely tailored for ourselves. Although point lists and protocols are a useful starting point, for the best results we need to respond with flexibility and adaptability. It's often the case that the points that are most sensitive are not to be found on any protocol or map.

Once we have found a tool, there are various ways to use it. The key variables are:

1. The speed of the press and release
2. The depth and pressure applied
3. The duration of the press
4. Any rotation or vibration

If you observe Dien Chan clinicians, you'll notice that everyone has slightly different techniques and ways of using the tools. This reflects their own style and approach. Generally speaking, though, if the press is fast and strong, it will be painful. The slower and lighter the pressure, the less pain and stimulation. If we're working on ourselves, it's much easier to find the ideal pressure. The rule of thumb I use is if there is any bracing against the point, then we are using too much pressure. The ideal is to find the "Goldilocks" zone, where the point is strong enough to be felt and affect a response but not so strong as to make one brace or contract.

If we have found a sensitive point it is useful to stay with this point for ten to thirty seconds, by which time there is usually a slight reduction in sensitivity, but pressing a point for five to ten seconds is often all that's necessary. There is no limit to how many points can be stimulated, so long as we keep in harmony with the setting and availability of each person. In Vietnam, treatments usually last between five and ten minutes. My own treatments are one to two hours.

Points can be stimulated without any intention, and their intrinsic effects can be relied upon. The body has its own wisdom and will take what is needed. This same principle is used in acupuncture with the harmonizing or even technique. However, in more nuanced situations it's helpful to know that one can stimulate a point with a range of intentions.

The two primary techniques are tonification and sedation—in other words, strengthening and fortifying—or to clear and dissipate. The main tonification technique I use is to press slowly, hold at a medium to strong pressure, and release slowly. The main reduction technique is to press quickly, hold at a light pressure, and use a slight vibration on the point. Although one needs to have some expertise in TCM diagnostics to utilize these techniques effectively on others, when it comes to self-massage, we can work intuitively if one or another point feels like it needs more or less pressure. The key is to keep listening and releasing as you go.

If you're looking to use Dien Chan for healing an illness, injury, or pain, I recommend consulting with a medical expert and starting

with the various point prescriptions available in the Dien Chan textbooks and apps. If you're seeking emotional regulation, soothing stress
and trauma, or working to transform mental-emotional patterns, I have
found the following points to be a useful place to start exploring:

1. 124, 34, 26 (on the forehead)
2. 16, 0, 14 (where the ear and face meet)
3. 61, 3, 37, 50 (by the nose and cheeks)
4. 7, 113, 17, 85, 127, 22 (around the mouth and chin)
5. 275, 283 (by the ear and eye)
6. 521, 126 (top and bottom of the centerline)

APPENDIX B

· ·

On Beauty
& Appearances

All the techniques and practices in this book have the side effect of acting as a natural face-lift. By boosting the microcirculation to the face, we help increase the health and luster of the skin. We can also help reduce any puffiness, discoloration, and wrinkling of the skin. As such, if desired, we can use Dien Chan to enhance our beauty. Not only does this have a positive effect on our health, but it can act as a natural alternative to cosmetic surgery and botox as well.

If we consider how important our facial expressivity is in both emotional self-regulation and in co-regulation and communication with others, we can conclude that anything that rigidifies our face will have a detrimental effect. There have been studies that show how the more botox is used, the less people are able to accurately read others' emotions, for they are effectively dampening the mimic muscles of the face and the mirroring aspects of communication. Notwithstanding that botox is the most potent neurotoxin known to humankind, there are many benefits for both our personal and social health if we opt for more natural methods of keeping up our appearances. There are, of course, exceptions, and cosmetic surgery can be miraculous in cases of injury and accident.

Dien Chan can act as a powerful technique in our beauty toolbox, but like any holistic approach, it's best framed within a comprehensive lifestyle. Diet and sleep are crucial, as are the products we choose to apply to our body, as they're very important for both our long-term health and the short-term effects. Generally speaking, I rarely use oils or creams on myself or in my treatments. The only exception is when the skin is especially dry, and particularly around the eyes. In this case I will use a small amount of serum. Dien Chan can be easily incorporated into a daily cosmetic routine. When we're bathing and cleaning our face and body, this is one of the easiest times to bring Dien Chan into our lives.

One of the secrets to warding off looking gray and haggard is improving our relationship with our emotions. If we are continuously angry or worried, our emotional expression will start to fix on our faces, creating patterned grooves and wrinkles. When we change our emotions, our face changes, too. The deeper level of emotional transformation, the clearer the change on the face. In some cases, old wrinkles can disappear if we transform old emotional patterns. Likewise, all the cosmetic treatments and face-lifts can do only so much if we are always frowning and stressing our face. When we feel peaceful, content, and naturally joyous, this brings out our most beautiful face. Therefore, using Dien Chan, meditation, and whatever emotional support is available to us will not only make us feel better inside but look better, too!

There is a massive industry that preys on people's insecurity and vanity. This is especially so for teenagers, and women in particular. Billions of dollars are made from the envy of lips, eyelashes, and skin. Often no matter how beautiful a person is, inside they will always feel like they're not beautiful enough. This drives many people to anxiety, panic, depression, body-shame, eating disorders, and suicide. There is even a new term—*snapchat dysmorphia*—that refers to how the popular social media platform is widely used alongside apps that change the appearance of one's face to be more beautiful. In turn, this creates the effect of always seeing the worst in oneself when looking in the mirror. Appearances can be very deceiving. It's for this reason, that tending to our emotional lives is only one part of the picture. Yes, feeling at home in our own skin is the foundation of emotional well-being. But we also need to change the way we see each other, to change our perception.

Specifically, if we judge one another only by appearance, we not only risk self-deception but also can fall prey to self-destructive ways of being and interaction. Instead, by withholding judgment toward others, we shift our mode of being from one of superficial seeing to a more truthful beholding. Behind each face lies much more than meets the eye. When we can behold other's in this way, we make space for all that is unknown in another person. Not only will this open stronger ties of connection and curiosity between each other, but we might also learn to appreciate the more implicit forms of beauty that are available in each face we see. This way of beholding beauty can form a mirror and double back on us. A joy shared is a joy doubled, as they say.

Whereas some might assume that holding any type of vanity is foolish, I think a wiser approach is to recognize that it's entirely natural to appreciate beauty in others and in ourselves. It's worth remembering that the root word of cosmetic comes from the Greek *cosmos,* which both refers to our world as a whole and also translates as "that which beautifies." When we appreciate beauty as an intrinsic part of life, we'll see the adornment of fashion and makeup as celebratory and life-affirming rather than superficial and meaningless.

Our capacity to appreciate beauty infuses our lives with meaning and purpose. For the mind that stops appreciating beauty and only sees utility and evolutionary advantage, quality of life, behavior, and health gradually diminish. We counteract this by consciously seeking out the beautiful, celebrating it, and adorning ourselves. This is the quite natural tendency we all have for an orientation toward beauty.

. . . .

The Descent, the Abyss & Dark Mother Energy

Loving Nature makes people protective of it. But what would happen if people believed that Nature loved them back? The relationship would become a sacred bond.

ROBIN WALL KIMMERER

The notion that we can enter a symbolic way of seeing the Earth, and that this can shift us into a state of feeling embedded within the Earth, as if held within a field of nurturing acceptance and love, is a process that is much easier to feel than to intellectually comprehend or rationally describe. Often, it's only when people have anomalous experiences that they will take seriously the notion that the Earth has symbolic dimensions, that the Earth conveys a presence, an undertone, and this interacts with our growth and personhood. This is an important challenge for us to explore individually, for if we can reframe our experience of the Earth as a place of inherent safety, rather than danger, our health and how we inhabit our bodies will be powerfully affected.

It will also extend out into how we relate to others and with the world-at-large.

It's very easy to raise objections to this notion that seem entirely valid—the extreme violence, suffering, and cruelty within nature being the most noticeable. There is a legitimate danger of idealizing nature as an entirely benevolent force, and in modern times this is seen in the simplification that everything natural must be good and everything synthetic must be bad. But nature has many faces; the symbolic Mother Earth is multivalent. The Earth carries layers and layers of meaning and implication, many of which are contradictory, and if we take any one strand, we can fall into interpretations of good and evil, or of framing life as entirely about survival or collaboration. This has direct implications for the idea that our bodies naturally want to heal if we can only harmonize with the healing resonance of nature.

In qigong, and in many indigenous understandings of Mother Earth, these objections are simply pointing to the destructive face of nature. How our modern culture relates to death has this tendency of framing the natural process of aging, of sustaining injury and illness, and of dying as being a failure of life, a failure of our bodies and our medicine. But, a relationship with the Earth as a mythical and symbolic place gives us an entirely different appreciation of life and death. Instead of seeing time as a flying arrow, we see time as a spinning wheel. This breaks the chain of seeing illness as only a trajectory of being broken to being fixed and changes how we place ourselves in time and space and how we make meaning of the tragedies and traumas of life. Health is not simply the absence of disease but rather an ongoing relational event that increases the vitality and beauty of our lives.

The destructive aspect of nature, which we can see in earthquakes, forest fires, tsunamis, and in nature as "red in tooth and claw," can easily be interpreted in our health as our bodies betraying us, which in turn necessitates a battle against illness, a war against our bodies and against nature. This draws us toward a reductionist view of our health and away from the holistic and interconnected reality. But, when we touch a human body, we are never just touching the hand or face, we are always touching the whole body. How we relate to our bodies mirrors how we relate to the Earth. In turn, this frames how we treat others in our family and community.

It's for this reason that in many traditional cultures there is great importance placed on rites and rituals that can illicit what I have termed *anomalous experiences*. These rituals are undertaken not only to deepen one's personal relationship with the Earth but also to develop a more subtle understanding of death. This deepening into subtlety is not only a matter of thought or language—although it does indeed change how we think and speak about the Earth—it's also a change in embodiment, how we stand and walk upon the Earth. There is a more visceral and immanent sense of the presence of death within our bodies and lives.

By contrast, when we feel separate from nature, there's a subtle displacement that occurs, a cultural dissociation and amnesia. Rituals and rites of passage strike a chord of remembrance in us, reminding us that we are just as much a part of the Earth as all the other plants, trees, and animals. And just like all this life around us, we will die one day, maybe sooner than we might expect, and this will feed the Earth. When we become too entranced by the idea of being separate from nature, we tend to feel disgusted by the idea that we might be food. We might even suppose, in the very back of our mind, that we're different from all the other life around us and that we can somehow escape our animal fate. This is an illusion, though. The way we relate to our death determines how well we nourish and feed the future ecology of life.

When we speak of the different dimensions of the Earth, in qigong this is explored by extending our felt sense of the body down into the depths of the ground. Like an elephant, we listen through our feet, and with some practice we start to feel the Earth as a layered being. The ground itself is just the face of the Earth, and we know there's a much greater biomass of life underneath the surface than up above. The soil is teeming with life, fungi, microbes, bacteria—a vast microscopic domain that remains largely unknown to us. Within the energetic and imaginal layers of the Earth, both creative and destructive forces percolate in different ways. It is important to recognize that there is a dark face of the Earth, which is sometimes called the death mother energy.

In our evolutionary past, we've been confronted with impossible decisions, and this death mother energy has been made manifest in the human realm. The choice to raise just one child or lose them all, which has been a harsh reality in the past, has affected our biology. This is one of the reasons why there is a deep taboo in many traditional cultures around the birth of twins. We all have in our mythical and genetic remembrance a wild twin who's been abandoned and forgotten. From an evolutionary perspective, this is one of the reasons why babies seek out and connect with other faces more than anything else, for if they can connect and bond to another person, they will be safe. It's one of the reasons why most people find babies so adorable.

However, the sad reality is that some people are orphaned from birth, and others grow up without the loving care of their mothers or caregivers. Being raised in an environment that doesn't embrace us has a profound effect on whether we see the world as inherently safe or dangerous. When we see only the danger in the world, this resonates with the destructive energy of the Earth. When we see the world as safe and as a source of nourishment and love, this awakens our pro-social nature and also gives us key advantages for long-term survival and flourishing.

The work of the evolutionary biologist David Sloan Wilson gives strong evidence that evolution is an interspecies process of collaboration, more than the hyper-Darwinist picture of competitive survival of the fittest. Taken to its logical end, this leads to the extreme narcissism and sociopathic tendencies that plague the power dynamics of society. The dark triad of narcissism, Machiavellianism, and psychopathy is rooted in developmental trauma just as much as any genetic cause—

or, in other words, the evils of the world stem from a perpetuation of trauma and a confused grasp of life. If we can see beyond our trauma, through a post-tragic lens, we realize that which gives us life and carries life onward wants us to feel embedded within the ecology of life as if embraced by a Mother Earth. This grounding of safety, acceptance, and love is spoken in a more-than-human tongue. And yet, it can be heard chiming out both from the ground beneath our feet and from within our bones. It communicates to us that our ancestry is not only human but also woven throughout the symbiosis of nature.

My conviction in this comes from an anomalous experience, rather than from thinking and reasoning. When I was on the cusp of adulthood, I had the good fortune of participating in a burial ritual, where, under the guidance and tutelage of elders and teachers, I spent a night buried underground. Although this might seem alarming to some, this kind of ritual is part of a long-standing tradition that aims to shift one's experience of the Earth. Whereas burial usually implies death, the ritual enacts a mythical encounter with the presence of death and, importantly, a resurrection into a new chapter in life. Although I will omit the details, I will say that whereas most people might assume that coming out of the Earth after a night buried alive would bring a sense of relief, this was not the case. Instead, rather than having a feeling of "at last, I'm free again," I felt an indescribable sense of contentment, as if I were bonded to the Earth in a nonhuman way—as if I was still within the Earth even after coming back up.

This sense of contentment was a beautiful and profound experience, like being permeated by a loving radiance and acceptance. The memory of it has sustained my spirit in times of adversity and has changed my relationship with death. It's left an imprint on me that gives me hope even in the face of the crushing statistics of impending doom. Although at the time I might not have explained it in these words, I see now that it had a profound effect on my nervous system and embodiment.

Our body mirrors and reflects the song of the Earth; it's a

resonant fractal jewel on Indra's Net. Because of this, the traditional rites and rituals that bring us into a deeper encounter with the mythical Earth specifically engage our body and physicality. In India and China, there's the hermitic tradition of retreating within forests, mountains, and caves. In Europe, there's the tradition of the wilderness vigil—sometimes called the vision quest—or the walkabout in Australia. In parts of Africa and the Mesoamerican traditions, there are rituals where one is buried underneath the Earth. All these rituals aim to bring us into deeper relationship and reciprocity with the process of death and the imaginal dimensions of the Earth—what is sometimes called the Soul of the Earth.

These rituals often share a pattern and rhythm, so much so that the mythologist Joseph Campbell labeled all the stories that accompany these rituals as the hero's journey, the mythical descent into the underworld. The hero with a thousand faces not only descends into the underworld and gambles with the lords and ladies of death, but he also returns with the heart of the beloved, a new way of being on the Earth.

One of my teachers, the embodiment expert Philip Shepherd, has drawn a remarkable similitude between the hero's journey and the process of being able to rest awareness within our body center, our abdomen. The descent into the underworld reflects the descent into the depths of our body. In the Chinese symbolic framing of the body, the abdomen is the Earth, and the head is the sky. What Shepherd shows us is that integrating our awareness throughout our body opens the world to us in a new way and at the same time gives us a way of being new to ourselves. In qigong this is called the marriage of heaven and Earth, an integration and coherence among our head, heart, and belly, which infuses life with pregnancy and creativity. Our own embodiment offers us an initiatory path toward greater embeddedment and connection to nature and toward discovering our true sovereign, that which serves the full ecology of life. From what we've explored throughout this book, we can see how being embodied through our abdomen and heart shifts our nervous system to a sense of safety and calm. Dien Chan aids us in the descent into our bodies, toward our origins.

Our personal history colors the sedimentary layers of our own body. Experiencing traumatic stress, great suffering, and brokenheartedness can make the journey into the underworld more precarious. We can awaken things that have been locked away in the dark dungeons of our being. What is sometimes called shadow work is undertaken by integrating the unique suffering of our personal stories and especially relates to our early childhood and formation of character. Because each person is unique in the way they inhabit their body, it's important to be flexible in the way we explore the deeper aspects of our embodiment. We need to find the most accessible entry point to make this inner journeying. If we know we have a lot of trauma to face, or have grown up in an insecure environment, it's highly recommended to find help from people or communities that have experience in trauma healing. We are never born alone, trauma always occurs in relationship between self and other, and healing trauma ultimately occurs through relational activity.

The hero's journey is not completed by simply delving into darkness or becoming embodied or individualized—it's not only a severance from the past. The crucial step is coming back to the community, to relate to the people and places around us with an open heart. As David Abram says, "We are human only in contact and conviviality with what is not human." Embodiment opens us to feeling the world, including all that is human and wild, through our bodies. This reciprocity with the world is, of course, supported when we return to a community that welcomes and accepts us.

But, even despite the confrontation with other people who aren't welcoming, or the nuances we carry in our emotional history, there is something universal about this pathway of integration among the face, heart, and belly. It brings us into a primordial encounter with the unknown, with our mortality, and this is a challenge all people share.

Learning to dance with this challenge is the great story and musicality we invoke through all lives.

The contemporary taboo surrounding these topics (death and hope) leads to the great cynicism we see in most adults. It is part of what has been termed the *meaning crisis*. Kastrup reflects that cynicism and fundamentalism are two sides of the same coin. In traditional cultures, one way of guarding against this is through the initiation rites that help carry teenagers into adulthood. This allows people to approach and wrestle with mortality in a way that won't maim us. Particularly in young men, and within the masculine part of ourselves, there is a rush toward death—toward the limits—and without the guidance of elders, this energy can become highly destructive to our communities. A look at the crisis of young male suicide reflects this. But, by coming into relationship with ourselves in a deeper sense—in an embodied and embedded sense—we can funnel this same energy toward birthing creativity, inspiration, and new life. How we go about this in modern times depends on what means are available to us. Although we might not have the wherewithal to undertake a longer and more immersive ritual, we all possess bodies; therefore, coming into touch with our bodies and the Earth in this mythical way is a viable and potent way of increasing health and vitality, both personally and in our immediate community.

It is my hope that Dien Chan and the self-care techniques presented in this book can offer us direct and accessible tools toward the discovery and rediscovery of the delight and deliciousness of being in our bodies and in this world. Being able to savor what the old Irish hero Finn MacCool called "the music of what is" averts all the tyrannical aspects of our person. Radiant contentment is a radical but life-affirming act. The downstream consequences will feed all our relationships.

Notes

INTRODUCTION.
HEALING FACES

1. Porges, "The Origins of Compassion." You can access the video to the lecture on YouTube.
2. Kirstin Konietzny, Boris Suchan, Nina Kreddig, Monika Hasenbring and Omar Chehadi, "Emotion Regulation and Pain: Behavioral and Neuronal Correlates: A Transdiagnostic Approach." Der Schmerz, October 2016, 30(5): 412–20. Also see Haines, *Pain is Really Strange*.
3. Baldwin, *As Much Truth As One Can Bear*.
4. Corbin, *Spiritual Body and Celestial Earth*.

1. THE ROOTS OF DIEN CHAN
FACIAL REFLEXOLOGY & QIGONG

1. Keown, *The Spark in the Machine*.
2. Van Nguyen and Pivar, *Fourth Uncle in the Mountain*.
3. Phillips, *Tai chi, Baguazhang and the Golden Elixir*.
4. Fruehauff, *Chinese Medicine in a Crises*.
5. Hsu, *Transmission of Chinese Medicine*.
6. Ochs, "The Liver and Kidneys Have the Same Source."
7. Palmer, *Qigong Fever*.

2. THE ROOTS OF STRESS & TRAUMA

1. Firdaus Dhabhar, *The Positive Effects of Stress.* You can access this TED Talk on YouTube.
2. Doidge, *The Brain That Changes Itself.*
3. Treleaven, *Trauma-Sensitive Mindfulness.*
4. Davis, *Light at the Edge of the World,* 138.
5. Sherman and Mehta, "Stress, Cortisol, and Social Hierarchy."
6. For a more in-depth history of trauma research see Nijenhuis, *The Trinity of Trauma.*
7. van der Kolk, "Posttraumatic Stress Disorder and the Nature of Trauma."
8. Levine, *In an Unspoken Voice.*
9. Maxwell, Merckelbach, Lilienfeld, and Lynn, "Treatment of Dissociation."
10. Ross, Joshi, and Currie, "Dissociative Experiences in the General Population."
11. Hrdy, *Mothers and Others.*
12. Nijenhuis, *The Trinity of Trauma.*
13. Nijenhuis, *The Trinity of Trauma.*
14. For a full breakdown of the absurdity of this argument, see Kastrup, *The Idea of the World.*
15. McGilchrist, *The Master and His Emissary.*
16. Kastrup, *The Idea of the World.*
17. Robinet, *The World Upside Down.*
18. Hart, *The Experience of God.*

3. THE ENERGETIC DYNAMIC
BETWEEN THE FACE & BODY

1. For an investigation into this, see Alex Scrimgeour, "What Is the Relationship between the Yi Jing (Classic of Change) with Chinese

Medicine?" BSc. Dissertation, College of Integrated Chinese Medicine, Kingston University, 2011.

2. Although implicit in many styles of qigong, these ideas have been greatly influenced by and stem from the work of the embodiment teacher Philip Shepherd. See Shepherd, *New Self, New World*.

3. Leighton, *Cultivating the Empty Field*.

4. THE GOLDEN ELIXIR & THE VAGUS NERVE

1. Yiming and Pregadio, *The Encyclopedia of Taoism*, vol. 1, 551–55.

2. Porges, *Pocket Guide to Polyvagal Theory*.

3. Monti, Porciello, Panasitin, and Aglioti, "The Inside of Me."

4. Robertson, *Vagus Nerve*.

5. Phillips, *Tai chi, Baguazhang and the Golden Elixir*.

6. Cheetham, *Imaginal Love*.

7. Cayley, *Rivers North of the Future*.

6. INDRA'S NET OF JEWELS

1. For further research into the role of ganying in ancient Chinese culture, see Sharf, *Coming to Terms with Chinese Buddhism;* and Le Blanc, *Huai-Nan Tzu*.

2. Ich'ing, *Shih-shuo Hsin-yu*.

3. Schneider, *A Beginner's Guide to Constructing the Universe*.

4. For a good overview of this research, see Kendall, *The Dao of Chinese Medicine*.

5. Neal, "Introduction to Neijing Classical Acupuncture."

6. Leighton, *Cultivating the Empty Field*.

7. Cleary, *Flower Ornament Scripture*.

8. Rovelli, *Helgoland*.

9. Sharma, *Interdependence*.

8. EMOTIONAL HISTORY

1. For an introduction into the current research and paradigm, see Barrett, *How Emotions Are Made*.
2. Rutger Bregman makes a strong case for revising these ideas in his recent book, *Human Kind: A Hopeful History*.
3. Ludwig and Welch, *Darwin's Other Dilemmas*.
4. Hrdy, *Mothers and Others*.
5. For a full breakdown of the inherent problems in this research, see chapter 1 of Lisa Feldman Barrett's work *How Emotions Are Made: The Secret Life of the Brain*.
6. Barrett, *How Emotions Are Made*.

10. EMOTIONS IN DIEN CHAN & CHINESE MEDICINE

1. Ni, *The Yellow Emporor's Classic of Medicine*, 95.
2. Ni, *The Yellow Emporor's Classic of Medicine*.
3. See Haines, *Trauma is Really Strange*. This series of science comic books is a wonderful resource for understanding the new paradigm surrounding embodiment, pain, and trauma.
4. Allan, *The Way of Water and Sprouts of Virtue*.
5. For a deeper look into these themes, see Zhang, *Human Dignity in Classical Chinese Philosophy;* and Csikszenthmihalyi, *Material Virtue*.
6. For a beautiful discussion on this theme, see the Perspectiva panel titled "The Post Tragic, with Marian Partington and Zak Stein." You can access the video on YouTube. See also the essay "From Pre-Tragic to Tragic to Post-Tragic Consciousness" by Marc Gafni, available at Academia.edu.
7. Alda, *If I Understood You, Would I Have This Look on My Face?*
8. Haines, *Trauma is Really Strange*.
9. Dante, *La Vita Nuov*. Barbara Reynolds, trans. Penguin, 1969.

10. Burbea, *Seeing That Frees.*

11. Pierre Teilhard de Chardin, *The Phenomenon of Man.*

12. THE TWO FACES OF BUDDHA

1. Shaw, *Courting the Wild Twin.*

2. See the 2016 Annual Blake Society Lecture, by Iain McGilchrist, available on YouTube.

3. Empson, *The Face of the Buddha.*

4. For more information on Ho'oponopono, see the work of Ilhaleakala Hew Len.

5. Robertson, *Vagus Nerve.*

13. EMBODIMENT & DISEMBODIMENT

1. Doidge, *The Brain That Changes Itself.*

2. Hoffman, *The Case Against Reality.*

3. Cayley, *Rivers North of the Future.*

4. Cranz, *Reorientations of Western Thought.* For further exploration, see Cheetham, *Imaginal Love.*

5. Illich, *In the Vineyard of the Text.* Also see John Vervaeke's work on Lectio Divina, available in Lecture 19 of his "Awakening from the Meaning Crisis" presentation. You can access the video on YouTube.

6. For insights into the concurrent changes in Chinese culture and medicine, see Goldschmidt, *The Evolution of Chinese Medicine.*

7. Nijenhuis, *The Trinity of Trauma.*

8. For detailed exploration into the distinctions between the embodied sovereign and the tyrant, see Shepherd, *New Self, New World.*

9. Hrdy, *Mothers and Others.*

10. Timothy Beardsworth, "A Sense of Presence: The Phenomenology of Certain Kinds of Visionary and Ecstatic Experience, Based on a Thousand Contemporary First-Hand Accounts" (RERC, 1977), quoted in Marshall, *Mystical Encounters with the Natural World.*

11. Rinpoche, *In Love with the World.*

12. Nijenhuis, *The Trinity of Trauma.*

13. Kastrup, *The Idea of the World.*

14. Hrdy, *Mothers and Others.*

15. Calaso, *The Celestial Hunter.*

16. Davis, *The Serpent and the Rainbow.*

14. DIEN CHAN FOR
EMBODIMENT & HOMECOMING

1. Liu, *Classical Chinese Medicine.*

15. RETURNING TO OUR SENSES

1. Moriarty, *Invoking Ireland.*

16. SILVER BRANCH PERCEPTION

1. Andreas Riener, "Information Injection below Conscious Awareness: Potential of Sensory Channels" (2011), quoted in Badenoch, *The Heart of Trauma.*

2. Moriarty, *Invoking Ireland.*

3. Charles Darwin, *Autobiographies* (New York; Penguin Classics, 2002), quoted in Moriarty, *Turtle Was Gone a Long Time.*

Bibliography

Abram, David. *The Spell of the Sensuous: Perception and Language in a More-Than-Human World.* New York: Vintage Books, 1997.

Adams, Joseph. "Reciprocal Innervation: A Modern Explanation of Neijing Branching Methodologies." *The American Acupuncturist Journal,* October 2006.

Alda, Alan. *If I Understood You, Would I Have This Look on My Face?* New York: Random House, 2017.

Allan, Sarah. *The Way of Water and Sprouts of Virtue.* Albany: State University of New York Press, 1997.

Atkins, Paul W., David Sloan Wilson, and Steven C. Hayes. *Prosocial: Using Evolutionary Science to Build Productive, Equitable, and Collaborative Groups.* Oakland, Calif.: New Harbinger, 2019.

Avens, Robert. *The New Gnosis: Hiedegger, Hillman, and Angels.* Thompson, Conn.: Spring Publications, 1984.

Badenoch, Bonnie. *The Heart of Trauma: Healing the Embodied Brain in the Context of Relationships.* New York: W. W. Norton and Company, 2018.

Baldwin, James. "As Much Truth as One Can Bear." *New York Times,* January 14, 1962.

Barfield, Owen. *Saving the Appearances: A Study in Idolatry.* New York: Harcourt, Brace, and World, 1957.

Barrett, Lisa Feldman. *How Emotions Are Made: The Secret Life of the Brain.* New York: Houghton Mifflin Harcourt, 2017.

Barret, Lewis, and Jeannette Haviland-Jones, eds. *The Handbook of Emotions,* 4th ed. New York: The Guilford Press, 2016.

Batchelor, Stephen. *The Art of Solitude.* New Haven, Conn.: Yale University Press, 2020.

Berman, Morris. *Wandering God: A Study in Nomadic Spirituality.* Albany: State University of New York Press, 2000.

Blackstone, Judith. *Belonging Here: A Guide for the Spiritually Sensitive Person.* Boulder, Colo.: Sounds True, 2002.

Bortoft, Henri. *Taking Appearances Seriously: The Dynamic Way of Seeing in Goethe and European Thought.* Edinburgh, UK: Floris Books, 2012.

Bortoft, Henri. *The Wholeness of Nature: Goethe's Way Towards a Science of Conscious Participation in Nature.* London: Lindesfarne Books, 1996.

Bregman, Rutger. *Human Kind: A Hopeful History.* London: Bloomsbury, 2019.

Bridges, Lillian. *Face Reading in Chinese Medicine.* Amsterdam: Elsevier, 2012.

Brine, Nathan. *The Taoist Alchemy of Wang Liping.* Vancouver: Dragon Gate Press, 2020.

Bruya, Brian, ed. *Effortless Attention: A New Perspective on the Cognitive Science of Attention and Action.* Cambridge, Mass.: MIT Press, 2010.

Burbea, Rob. *Seeing That Frees: Meditations on Emptiness and Dependant Arising.* West Ogwell: Hermes Amara, 2014.

Burgs. *Living Dharma: The Flavour of Liberation,* vol. 4. Self-Published, 2017.

Calasso, Roberto. *The Celestial Hunter.* London: Allen Lane, 2020.

———. *Ka: Stories of the Mind and Gods of India.* New York: Vintage, 1996.

Callard, Agnes. *Aspiration: The Agency of Becoming.* Oxford: Oxford University Press, 2018.

Carey, John, trans. *The Ever-New Tongue (In Tenga Bithnua): The Text in the Book of Lismore.* Turnhout: Brepols Publishers, 2018.

Cayley, David. *Rivers North of the Future: The Testament of Ivan Illich.* Toronto: House of Anansi Press, 2005.

Chang, Garma C. C. *The Buddhist Teaching of Totality: The Philosophy of Hwa Yen Buddhism.* University Park: Pennsylvania State University Press, 1971.

Cheetham, Tom. *All the World an Icon: Henry Corbin and the Angelic Function of Beings.* Berkeley, Calif.: North Atlantic Books, 2012.

———. *Imaginal Love: The Meanings of Imagination in Henry Corbin and James Hillman.* Thompson, Conn: Spring Publications, 2015.

Chen, Nancy. *Breathing Spaces: Qigong, Psychiatry and Healing in China.* New York: Columbia University Press, 2003.

Ching-Yun, Li. *Master.* Rochester, Vt.: Healing Arts Press, 2002.

Cleary, Thomas. *The Flower Ornament Scripture: A Translation of the Avatamsaka Sutra.* Boulder, Colo.: Shambhala, 1984.

Corbin, Henry. *Alone With the Alone: Creative Imagination in the Sufism of Ibn 'Arabi.* Princeton, N.J.: Princeton University Press, 1969.

———. *Jung, Buddhism, and the Incarnation of Sophia.* Rochester, Vt.: Inner Traditions, 2019.

———. *Spiritual Body and Celestial Earth: From Mazdean Iran to Shi'ite Iran.* Princeton, N.J.: Princeton University Press, 1977.

Craig, A. G. *How do you Feel? An Interoceptive Moment with your Neurobiological Self.* Princeton, N.J.: Princeton University Press, 2015.

Cranz, F. Edward. *Reorientations of Western Thought from Antiquity to the Renaissance.* Burlington Vt.: Ashgate/Variorum, 2006.

Csikszentmihalyi, Mark. *Material Virtue: Ethics and Body in Early China.* Leiden: Brill, 2004.

Currivan, Jude. *The Cosmic Hologram: In-Formation at the Centre of Creation.* Rochester, Vt.: Inner Traditions, 2017.

Darcia, Narvaez. *Neurobiology and the Development of Human Morality: Evolution, Culture, and Wisdom.* New York: W. W. Norton and Company, 2014.

Davis, Wade. *Light at the Edge of the World: A Journey through the Realm of Vanishing Cultures.* Vancouver: Douglas and McIntyre, 2007.

———. *The Serpent and the Rainbow.* New York: Harper Collins, 1986.

Doidge, Norman. *The Brain That Changes Itself.* London: Penguin, 2008.

Eagleman, David. *Livewired: The Inside Story of the Ever-Changing Brain.* Edinburgh: Canongate Books, 2020.

Eisler, Riane, and Douglas P. Fry. *Nurturing Our Humanity: How Domination and Partnership Shape Our Brains, Lives, and Future.* Oxford: Oxford University Press, 2019.

Ekman, Paul, and Wallace V. Friesen. *Unmasking the Face: A Guide to Recognising Emotions from Facial Expressions.* San Jose, Calif.: Malor Books, 2003.

Empson, William. *The Face of the Buddha.* Oxford: Oxford University Press, 2016.

Fernández-Dols, José-Miguel, and James A. Russel, eds. *The Science of Facial Expression.* Oxford: Oxford University Press, 2017.

Ferrer, Jorge N., and Jacob H. Sherman. *The Participatory Turn: Spirituality, Mysticism, Religious Studies.* Albany, N.Y.: SUNY Press, 2008.

Fuller, Robert C. *Wonder: From Emotion to Spirituality.* Chapel Hill, N.C.: University of North Carolina Press, 2006.

Fruehauff, Heiner. "Chinese Medicine in a Crises: Science, Politics and the Making of 'TCM.'" *Journal of Chinese Medicine,* October 1999.

Gafni, Marc, and Kristina Kincaid. *A Return to Eros: The Radical Experience of Being Fully Alive.* Dallas: BenBella Books, 2017.

Goldschmidt, Asaf. *The Evolution of Chinese Medicine: Song Dynasty, 960–1200.* Abingdon, Oxford: Routledge, 2011.

Habib, Navaz. *Activate your Vagus Nerve.* Berkeley, Calif.: Ulysses Press, 2019.

Haines, Steve. *Pain is Really Strange.* London: Singing Dragon, 2015.

———. *Touch is Really Strange.* London: Singing Dragon, 2021.

———. *Trauma is Really Strange.* London: Singing Dragon, 2016.

Hamar, Imre, *Reflecting Mirrors: Perspectives on Huayan Buddhism.* Weisbaden: Harrassowitz Verlag, 2007.

Hart, David Bentley. *The Experience of God: Being, Consciousness, Bliss.* New Haven, Conn.: Yale University Press, 2013.

Hinrichs, T. J. *Chinese Medicine and Healing: An Illustrated History.* Cambridge, Mass.: Harvard University Press, 2012.

Hjortsjö, Carl-Herman. *Man's Face and Mimic Language.* Lund, Sweden: Studentlitteratur, 1969.

Hoffman, Donald D. *The Case Against Reality: How Evolution Hid the Truth from Our Eyes.* New York: Penguin, 2019.

Holman, C. T. *Treating Emotional Trauma with Chinese Medicine*. London: Singing Dragon, 2017.

Hrdy, Sarah Blaffer. *Mothers and Others: The Evolutionary Origins of Mutual Understanding*. Cambridge, Mass.: Harvard University Press, 2011.

Hsu, Elisabeth. *The Transmission of Chinese Medicine*. Cambridge, UK: Cambridge University Press, 1999.

Hunt, Maurice. *The Divine Face in Four Writers: Shakespeare, Dostoyevsky, Hesse, C.S. Lewis*. London: Bloomsbury Academic, 2016.

Iacoboni, Marco. *Mirroring People: The Science of Empathy and How We Connect with Others*. London: Picador, 2008.

Ich'ing, Liu. *Shih-shuo Hsin-yu*. Translated by Richard B. Mather. Ann Arbor: University of Michigan, 2002.

Illich, Ivan. *In the Vineyard of the Text: A Commentary to Hugh's Didascalicon*. Chicago, Ill.: University of Chicago Press, 1996.

Jullien, François. *Detour and Access: Strategies of Meaning in China and Greece*. Translated by Sophie Hawkes, New York: Zone Books, 2004.

Kastrup, Bernardo. *The Idea of the World: A Multidisciplinary Argument for the Mental Nature of Reality*. Alresford: Iff Books, 2019.

Keown, Daniel. *The Spark in the Machine: How the Science of Acupuncture Explains the Mysteries of Western Medicine*. London: Singing Dragon, 2014.

Kespi, Jean-Marc. *Acupuncture: From Symbol to Clinical Practice*. Seattle: Eastland Press, 2012.

Khun, Philip A. *Soulstealers: The Chinese Sorcery Scare of 1768*. Cambridge, Mass.: Harvard University Press, 1990.

Kohn, Eduardo. *How Forests Think: Toward an Anthropology Beyond the Human*. Berkeley: University of California Press, 2013.

Korn, Leslie E. *Rhythms of Recovery: Trauma, Nature, and the Body*. Abingdon: Routledge, 2013.

Kripal, Jeffery J. *The Flip: Who You Really Are and Why It Matters*. New York: Penguin, 2020.

Lachman, Gary. *Lost Knowledge of the Imagination*. Edinburgh, UK: Floris Books, 2017.

Lakoff, George, and Mark Johnson. *Philosophy in the Flesh: The Embodied Mind and Its Challenge to Western Thought*. New York: Basic Books, 1999.

Lanius, Ulrick F., Sandra L. Paulsen, and Frank M. Corrigan, eds. *Neurobiology and Treatment of Traumatic Dissociation: Toward and Embodied Self.* New York: Springer Publishing, 2014.

Le Blanc, Charles. *Huai-Nan Tzu: Philosophical Synthesis in Early Han Thought. The Idea of Resonance (Kan-Ying)*. Hong Kong: Hong Kong University Press, 1985.

Lefferts, Marshall. *Cosmometry: Exploring the HoloFractal Nature of the Cosmos*. Santa Cruz, Calif.: Cosmometria Publishing, 2019.

Leighton, Taigen Dan. *Cultivating the Empty Field: The Silent Illumination of Zen Master Hongzhi*. Clarendon, Vt.: Tuttle, 2000.

Levine, Peter. *In an Unspoken Voice: How the Body Releases Trauma and Restores Goodness*. Berkeley, Calif.: North Atlantic Books, 2010.

Lewis, Mark Edward. *The Construction of Space in Early China*. Albany, N.Y.: SUNY Press, 2012.

Lewontin, R. C. *Biology as Ideology: The Doctrine of DNA*. Toronto: House of Anansi Press, 1991.

Liu, Han Wen. *Chan Mi Gong: Chinese Meditation for Health*. Translated by Gabriel Weiss, Henry A. Buchtel, and Sabine Wilms. Montery, Calif: Victoria Press, 2009.

Liu, Lihong. *Classical Chinese Medicine*. Translated by Gabriel Weiss, Hanry A. Buchtel, and Sabine Wilms. Hong Kong: The Chinese University Press, 2019.

Liu, Xun. *Daoist Modern: Innovation, Lay Practice, and the Community of Inner Alchemy in Republican Shanghai*. Cambridge, Mass.: Harvard University, 2009.

Lomax, Michael L. *A Light Warrior's Guide to High Level Energy Healing: Medical Qigong and A Shaman's Healing Vision*. Thayer, Mo.: Spirit Way Publications, 2000.

Ludwig, Robert J., and Martha G. Welch. "Darwin's Other Dilemmas and the Theoretical Roots of Emotional Connection." *Frontline Psychology Journal,* April 12 2019.

Lyman, Monty. *The Remarkable Life of the Skin: An Intimate Journey Across Our Surface*. London: Black Swan, 2020.

Marshall, Paul. *Mystical Encounters with the Natural World: Experiences and Explanations*. Oxford: Oxford University Press, 2005.

Maté, Gabor. *In the Realm of Hungry Ghosts: Close Encounters with Addiction*. Berkeley, Calif.: North Atlantic Books, 2011.

Maxwell, Reed, Harald Merckelbach, Scott Lilienfeld, and Steven Lynn. "The Treatment of Dissociation: The State of the Science and Practice," chapter 13 in *Evidence Based Psychotherapy: The State of the Science and Practice*. Hoboken, N.J.: Wiley-Blackwell, 2018, 329–61.

McGilchrist, Iain. *The Master and His Emissary: The Divided Brain and the Making of the Western World*. New Haven, Conn.: Yale University Press, 2010.

Meyer, Kuno, trans. *The Voyage of Bran*. Cambridge, Ontario: In Parentheses Publications, 2000.

Miller, Dan, and Tim Cartmell. *Xing Yi Nei Gong: Xing Yi Health Maintenance and Internal Development*. West Fork, Ark.: High View Publications, 2004.

Moeller, Hans-Georg, and Andrew K. Whitehead. *Imagination: Cross-Cultural Philosophical Analysis*. London: Bloomsbury Academic, 2018.

Monti, Aessandro, Gioseppina Porciello, Maria Serena Panasiti, and Salvatore Maria Aglioti. "The Inside of Me: Interoceptive Constraints on the Concept of Self in Neuroscience and Clinical Psychology." *Psychological Research,* May 2021.

Moriarty, John. *Invoking Ireland: Ailia Iath N-hErend*. Dublin: Lilliput, 2005.

———. *Turtle Was Gone a Long Time,* vol. 2. Dublin: Lilliput, 1997.

———. *A Hut at the Edge of the Village*. Edited by Martin Shaw. Dublin: Lilliput, 2021.

Nachmanovitch, Stephen. *The Art of Is: Improvising as a Way of Life*. Novato: New World Library, 2019.

Neal, Edward. "Introduction to Neijing Classical Acupuncture." *Journal of Chinese Medicine* 100: October 2012.

Ni, Maoshing, trans. *The Yellow Emporor's Classic of Medicine*. Boston: Shambhala, 1995.

Nicholson, Daniel J. *Everything Flows: A Processual Philosophy of Biology*. Oxford: Oxford University Press, 2018.

Nijenhuis, Ellert. *The Trinity of Trauma: Ignorance, Fragility, and Control. The Evolving Concept of Trauma/The Concept and Facts of Dissociation in Trauma*. Göttingen: Vandenhoeck and Ruprecht, 2015.

Ochs, Shelley. "The Liver and Kidneys Have the Same Source: Knowing the Theory, Realising the Doctrine." *Journal of Chinese Medicine,* October 2005.

O'Donoghue, Brendan, ed. *A Moriarty Reader: Preparing for Early Spring*. Dublin: Lilliput, 2012.

Olsen, Stuart Alve. *Qigong Teachings of a Daoist Immortal: The Eight Essential Exercises of Master Li Ching-yun*. Rochester, Vt.: Healing Arts Press, 2002.

Pallasmaa, Juhani. *The Eyes of the Skin: Architecture and the Senses*. Hoboken, N.J.: Wiley, 1996.

Palmer, David. *Qigong Fever: Body, Science and Utopia in China*. London: Hurst, 2007.

Palmer, David, and Liu Xun. *Daoism in the Twentieth Century: Between Eternity and Modernity*. Berkeley: University of California Press, 2012.

Paper, Jordan D. *The Dieties Are Many: A Polytheistic Theology*. Albany, N.Y.: SUNY Press, 2005.

Phillips, Scott Park. *Possible Origins: A Cultural History of Chinese Martial Arts, Theater, and Religion*. Boulder, Colo.: Angry Baby Books, 2016.

———. *Tai chi, Baguazhang and the Golden Elixir: Internal Martial Arts before the Boxer Uprising*. Boulder, Colo.: Angry Baby Books, 2019.

Porges, Stephen W. "The Origins of Compassion: A phylogenic perspective." Lecture given at the Science of Compassion Convention at Stanford University in July 2012. You can access the video on YouTube.

———. *The Pocket Guide to Polyvagal Theory: The Transformative Power of Feeling Safe*. New York: W. W. Norton and Company, 2017.

———. *Polyvagal Theory: Neurophysiological Foundations of Emotions, Attachment, Communication, Self-Regulation.* New York: W. W. Norton and Company, 2011.

Prechtel, Martin. *Long Life, Honey in the Heart: A Story of Eloquence and Initiation on the Shores of a Mayan Lake.* New York: Tarcher and Putnam, 2001.

Pregadio, Fabrizio. *Taoist Internal Alchemy: An Anthology of Neidan Texts.* Mount View, Calif.: Golden Elixir Press, 2019.

———. *The Way of the Golden Elixir: An Introduction to Taoist Alchemy.* Mount View, Calif.: Golden Elixir Press, 2019.

Ridley, Matt. *The Origins of Virtue.* New York: Viking, 1996.

Rinpoche, Yongey Mingyur. *In Love with the World: What a Monk Can Teach You About Living from Nearly Dying.* Monument, Colo.: Bluebird, 2021.

Robertson, Caroline. *Vagus Nerve.* Self-Published, 2020.

Robinet, Isabelle. *The World Upside Down: Essays on Taoist Internal Alchemy.* Mount View, Calif.: Golden Elixir Press, 2011.

Roche, Lorin. *The Radiance Sutras: 112 Gateways to the Yoga of Wonder and Delight.* Boulder, Colo.: Sounds True, 2014.

Rosin, Ross. *Heart-Shock: Diagnosis and Treatment of Trauma with Shen-Hammer and Classical Chinese Medicine.* London: Singing Dragon, 2018.

Ross, Colin A., Shaun Joshi, and Raymond Currie. "Dissociative Experiences in the General Population." *Hospital and Community Psychiatry* 42(3) (1990): 297–301.

Rovelli, Carlo. *Helgoland.* New York: Penguin, 2021.

Santangelo, Paulo, ed. *Love, Hatred, and Other Passions: Questions and Themes on Emotions in Chinese Civilization.* Leiden: Brill, 2006.

Santangelo, Paulo. *From Skin to Heart: Perceptions of Emotions and Bodily Sensations in Traditional Chinese Culture.* Weisbaden: Harrassowitz Verlag, 2006.

Schneider, Michael S. *A Beginner's Guide to Constructing the Universe: The Mathematical Archetypes of Nature, Art, and Science.* New York: Avon Books, 1995.

Sharf, Robert H. *Coming to Terms with Chinese Buddhism: A Reading of the Treasure Store Treatise.* Honolulu: University of Hawaii Press, 2002.

Sharma, Kriti. *Interdependence: Biology and Beyond.* New York: Fordham University Press, 2015.

Shaw, Martin. *Courting the Wild Twin.* Hartford, Vt.: Chelsea Green, 2020.

———. *Snowy Tower: Parzival and the Wet, Black, Branch of Language.* Ashland, Oreg.: White Cloud Press, 2004.

Shepherd, Philip. *New Self, New World: Recovering Our Senses in the 21st Century.* Berkeley, Calif.: North Atlantic Books, 2010.

———. *Radical Wholeness: The Embodied Present and the Ordinary Grace of Being.* Berkeley, Calif.: North Atlantic Books, 2017.

Sherman, Gary D., and Pranjal H. Mehta. "Stress, Cortisol, and Social Hierarchy." *Current Opinion in Psychology* 33 (June 2020): 227–32.

Shi Zi, Yin. *Tranquil Sitting: A Taoist Journal on Meditation and Chinese Medical Qigong.* Translated by Shifu Hwang and Cheney Crow. London: Singing Dragon, 2012.

Sieff, Daniela F. *Understanding and Healing Emotional Trauma: Conversations with Pioneering Clinicians and Researchers.* Abingdon, Oxford: Routledge, 2017.

Slingerland, Edward. *Mind and Body in Early China: Beyond Orientalism and the Myth of Holism.* Oxford: Oxford University Press, 2019.

Smith, Frederick M. *The Self Possessed: Diety and Spirit Possession in South Asian Literature and Civilisation.* New York: Columbia University Press, 2006.

Stein, Zachary. *Education in a Time between Worlds: Essays on the Future of Schools, Technology and Society.* Bright Alliance, 2019.

Tanaka, Koji, ed. *The Moon Points Back.* Oxford: Oxford University Press, 2015.

Teilhard de Chardin, Pierre. *The Phenomenon of Man.* London: Collins, 1959.

Thich Naht Hanh. *How to Love.* Berkeley, Calif: Parallax Press, 2015.

———. *The Miracle of Mindfulness.* Boston: Beacon Press, 1975.

Treleaven, David A. *Trauma-Sensitive Mindfulness: Practices for Safe and Transformative Healing.* New York: W. W. Norton and Company, 2018.

Turner, Edith. *Communitas: The Anthropology of Collective Joy.* London: Palgrave Macmillan, 2012.

Vagal, Thomas. "What Is It Like to Be a Bat?" *The Philosophical Review* 83, no. 4 (1974).

van der Kolk, Bessel. *The Body Keeps the Score: Mind, Brain, and Body in the Transformation of Trauma*. New York: Penguin, 2015.

——. "Posttraumatic Stress Disorder and the Nature of Trauma." *Dialogues in Clinical Neuroscience* 2, no. 1 (2000): 7–22.

Van Nguyen, Quang, and Marjorie Pivar. *Fourth Uncle in the Mountain: A Memoir of a Barefoot Doctor in Vietnam*. New York: St. Martin's Press, 2004.

Varela, Francisco J., Evan Thompson, and Eleanor Rosch. *The Embodied Mind: Cognitive Science and the Human Experience*. Cambridge, Mass.: MIT Press, 2017

Wang, Fengyi. *Discourse on Transforming Inner Nature: Hua Xing Tan*. Translated by Johan Hausen and Jonas T. Akers. Purple Cloud Press, 2018.

Wang, Ju-Yi, and Jason D. Robertson. *Applied Channel Theory*. Seattle: Eastland Press, 2008.

Wen, Benebell. *The Tao of Craft: Fu Talismans and Casting Sigils in the Eastern Esoteric Tradition*. Berkeley, Calif.: North Atlantic Books, 2016.

Wilms, Sabine, trans. *Twelve Characters: A Transmission of Wang Fengyi's Teachings*. Corbet, Oreg.: Happy Goat Productions, 2014.

Wilson, David Sloan. *This View of Life: Completing the Darwinian Revolution*. Yang, Sōetsu. *The Unknown Craftsman: A Japanese Insight into Beauty*. New York: Alfred A. Knopf. 2019.

Yanagi, Sōetsu. *The Unknown Craftsman: A Japanese Insight into Beauty*. New York: Kodansha International, 1972.

Yiming, Liu, and Fabrizio Pregadio, trans. *The Encyclopedia of Taoism*, vol. 1. Abingdon, Oxford: Routledge, 2008.

Yuen, Jeffrey C. *San Shen Qi Ling: 3 Spirits and 7 Souls*. Worcester, Mass.: New England School of Acupuncture, 2005.

Yunkaporta, Tyson. *Sand Talk: How Indigenous Thinking Can Save the World*. Melbourne: Text Publishing, 2019.

Zarins, Uldins. *Anatomy of Facial Expression*. New York: Anatomy Next, 2017.

Zhang, Qianfan. *Human Dignity in Classical Chinese Philosophy: Confucianism, Mohism, and Daoism*. London: Palgrave Macmillan, 2016.

Acknowledgments

The inspiration for this book has come from many directions, and the journey of writing it has been helped and motivated by many people. Initially, my reason for starting this book was to share the remarkable practice of Dien Chan with my clients and those who are interested in learning the deeper aspects of Dien Chan. The process itself has also helped me integrate and clarify the many teachings with which I have been blessed.

To the people who most nourish and support me—my dear family and parents—thank you. Thank you to my brother Dan who has greatly helped in giving feedback on the text.

To the people who have taught me and guided me into the healing arts—my clients, teachers, and friends—thank you.

In the realms of Chinese medicine, qigong, and meditation, I am most indebted to Tai H. Long—your calm presence, skill, and humor have been a continuous inspiration. Thank you.

Thank you to the qigong master Michael Lomax, for initiating me into Jing Dong Gong, and for all the wondrous experiences in dreamtime.

Thank you to the tai chi chuan master Murray Douglas, for gifting me with a lifelong practice that continues to unfold and amaze. Thank you to the grandmaster Sifu Yeung Ma Lee, for both preserving and innovating this wonderful art.

Thank you to Burgs for all the support, teachings, and imparted wisdom—I have so much gratitude and love for you and all that you have done for my family and the greater community.

Thank you to the Zen teacher Thich Nhat Hanh.

In the realms of embodiment and story, two great teachers and wandering troubadours have conjured new people out of me—Dr. Martin Shaw, thank you for waking us up and showing us there are always new possibilities, even when everything seems finished. To Philip Shepherd, thank you for your revelatory writing and the gentle guidance into the unknown.

Thank you to all the teachers who have shared their time and energy with me—Ram Chatlani, Manola Cetina, C. T. Holman, John and Angie Hicks, Michael Phoenix, Jane Blake, Richard Birtschinger, S. J. Marshall, Master Zhongxian Wu, Ajahn Luangta, Jason Robertson, Donald Rubbo, Master Lam Kam Chuen, Professor Truong Thin, Andrew Nugent-Head, Tim Sullivan, May Raksakan, Richard Tan, Steve Haines, Simon Tafler, Wu De and Shen Su, Pichest and Aon Boonthumme, Glynda in Samui and Martín Prechtel.

Thank you to all the teachers who have unbeknown to them helped my life and this book. Of significance—John Moriarty, David Abram, Brian Bates, Quang Van Nguyen, Hazrat Inayat Khan, Tom Cheetham, Jeffrey Yuen, Liu Lihong, Lisa Feldman Barrett, Iain McGilchrist, Peter Levine, Heiner Fruehof, Ellert Nijenhuis, Dr. Edward Neal, Scott Park Phillips, Stephen Porges, Daniella Sieff, Dr. Jerry Alan Johnson, Lillian Bridges, Kriti Sharma, and Zachary Stein. Without your creativity this book would be hollow.

In the spa, health, and wellness communities, I am indebted to the faith and support given to me by Clare Beardson, who introduced me to Hong Kong and the old-time joie de vivre of the Mandarin Oriental. Also, a special thanks to John and Karina Stewart, Karen Aleksich, Emmanuell Bellec, and Suzi Scott.

Much of this book has been written in my downtime working at Ulpotha in Sri Lanka, Kamalaya in Thailand, the Mandarin Oriental in Morocco, and Nihi Sumba in Indonesia, so I offer a dept of gratitude to these healing spaces for gifting me the perfect environment for writing. Despite the devastating and world-twisting effects of the 2020 pandemic, without this curse I would not have had the dedicated time to finish this book, so thank you to SARS-CoV-2 for this creative hastening. Thank you for the global wake-up call, may we awaken from our slumber.

In the great task of making a book come alive, thank you to Stephen Brough, Charlie Viney, and Rupert Sheldrake—your invaluable advice has steered me well. Thank you to Daniel Reid, for both your advice and commendation and for your own incredible books. Thank you to Jon Graham and all the good people at Inner Traditions • Bear & Company. Thank you for the most wonderful illustrations, Kat Lowe! May your brush never run dry. Thank you to Merlin Sheldrake for the hot tips and to Mariko Bangerter for the kind help and dialogue.

Finally, thank you to the kind people who welcomed me and taught me in Vietnam. Thank you to Madame Nguyen Viet Nga, for gifting me your acupressure and meditation wisdom. Thank you to Martin Gelardo, for being in the right place at the right time and for your living example of a real barefoot doctor. Thank you to Wendy Stein, for your friendship and showing me Saigon. Thank you to Alex and Hong Gabriel for hosting me in Ho Chi Minh City and for making such vital introductions to the Institute of Traditional Vietnamese Medicine and to the Dien Chan master Tran Dung Thang. Thank you, Dr. Tran, for such boundless kindness, generosity, and soul. May your memory continue to inspire and relieve the suffering of others.

Thank you and a thousand blessings to Professor Bui Cuoc Chau, his family, and the healing community at the Viet Y Dao Centre. May your achievements keep reverberating through and healing this world. Thank you to the teacher and master practitioner Bui Minh Tri, for your kindness and good humor.

For any mistakes, omissions, or confusion caused by this book, I take full responsibility. For all the shortcomings and imperfections, please forgive me; I am truly sorry and continue to be awed by and in deep gratitude to the greater beings who walk out ahead of us. Our faces are always darkened by the shadows of the greater angels of our being. May their bright presence illuminate our path forward out of suffering and confusion.

Index

About the Author

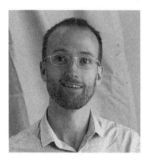 ALEX SCRIMGEOUR is a licensed acupuncturist and massage therapist based in London. He earned a bachelor of science degree in acupuncture and a diploma in Tui-Na massage from the College of Integrated Chinese Medicine, the United Kingdom's largest acupuncture college. After receiving his degree, Alex completed a six-week clinical internship at Vietnam's largest teaching hospital, the Institute of Traditional Vietnamese Medicine in Ho Chi Minh City, where he formed relationships with some of the country's leading acupuncturists and massage therapists. He has studied extensively with Trần Dũng Thắng, Bùi Minh Trí, and other master Dien Chan clinicians at the Việt Y Đạo Center.

More recently, Alex has been developing innovative treatments to help people suffering from PTSD, anxiety, and stress disorders. He has created tailored qigong teachings and tea ceremony for Khiron House, a leading trauma center in Oxfordshire. He also provides treatments and teaches at many of the leading spas and wellness centers around the world, including the Mandarin Oriental Hotel in Hong Kong.

For more on Alex Scrimgeour's practice and treatments visit his website, **alexscrimgeour.com.**

For an online course Alex created as a companion to this book, visit **sensoryselfcare.com.**